THE
Soul
WORKOUT

Getting and Staying Spiritually Fit

By Helen H. Moore

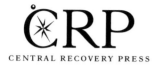

CENTRAL RECOVERY PRESS

Central Recovery Press (CRP) is committed to publishing exceptional materials addressing addiction treatment, recovery, and behavioral health care, including original and quality books, audio/visual communications, and Web-based new media. Through a diverse selection of titles, it seeks to impact the behavioral health care field with a broad range of unique resources for professionals, recovering individuals, and their families.

For more information, visit www.centralrecoverypress.com.

Central Recovery Press, Las Vegas, NV 89129
© 2010 by Central Recovery Press, Las Vegas, NV

ISBN-13: 978-0-9799869-8-7
ISBN-10: 0-9799869-8-2

16 15 14 13 12 11 10   2 3 4 5

Publisher: Central Recovery Press
            3371 N Buffalo Drive
            Las Vegas, NV 89129

AUTHOR'S NOTE: This is a true story of my life and my recovery experiences recounted to the best of my memory. All opinions expressed are my own. All names have been changed to protect privacy and anonymity. Characters, places, and incidents are composites. Any resemblance to actual persons, living or dead, is entirely unintentional.

Cover design and interior by Sara Streifel, Think Creative Design

DEDICATED TO THE MEN AND
WOMEN OF MY HOME GROUP,
TO MY SPONSOR, N J,
AND TO KIM CATALANO.

CONTENTS

ACKNOWLEDGMENTS

With gratitude to Stuart Smith, whose wholehearted dedication to the cause of recovery gave me the opportunity to share my "experience, strength, and hope" in these pages. His vision and commitment have helped many in recovery.

I would like to thank my editor, Nancy Schenck. Without her willingness to embrace my ideas and her kindness, insight, diligence, and expertise, this book would have remained merely an idea in its author's head.

Thank you to Daniel Kaelin, Valerie Killeen, and Dan Mager, my industrious colleagues at Central Recovery Press, for their patience and hard work.

INTRODUCTION

At a meeting of my home group one morning, I looked around at all the members. These were the strangers whose kindness I had once depended upon for my life, the strangers who had become my friends and my teachers. In this room, I heard an old-timer say, "Put back your shopping cart." I heard a member say, "Don't tell me how much you love your kid; just pay your child support." I heard a woman say, "Do good and don't get caught." I also heard, "Making amends means standing in their driveway with their money in your hand."

This dingy church hall, I realized, was the gym that we came to in order to exercise our spirituality, taking time every day for what I came to call "The Soul Workout."

I was sitting in that hall listening to the others because I was trying to save my life. I have the chronic, progressive, and fatal brain disease of addiction, which affects me physically, mentally, emotionally, and spiritually. In recovery, I began to get better in this order:

* First, physically, as substances left my system;

* Then, mentally and emotionally, as the toxins cleared my brain and I received unwavering support from my twelve-step fellowship;

* And finally, I began to recover spiritually.

As I did, I began to realize that each day I had spent in my active disease was a day in which I took my soul in both hands and shredded it. Toward the end of my active addiction, there was very little left of it, and I was living my life close to the animal level.

An addict is, practically by definition, almost completely consumed by self: self-will, self-centeredness, self-pity, self-importance, and self-hate. Spirituality is the primary means I have to break that obsession with self and put the emphasis where it belongs—on self in service to others. This change of emphasis breaks the compulsion and obsession at the heart of addiction, replacing the self-obsession with connectedness, fellowship, and love.

Service to others can take many forms, but it often starts when an addict simply reaches out to help other addicts. A smile for a newcomer in recovery, a hug for a new friend, a compliment offered sincerely, or a word of encouragement—these are small but important beginnings. I grow in spirit by being helpful, kind, and loving to others, and by treating them as I would want to be treated. I know this sounds so simple as to be trite, but, as an addict in active addiction, I was one of the most self-centered creatures imaginable, selfish beyond even thinking of performing these simple acts of basic human decency.

As I begin to reenter the mainstream of life, I extend this attitude of service to others, inside my fellowship and out. Paradoxically, I realize that the rewards I reap by extending myself to others will be ever greater, my spiritual "armor" ever stronger, the more I do for them. That is the philosophy behind this book, and it can work for anyone, whether inside or outside a recovery program.

In my active addiction, each lie I told, each cynical manipulation I engaged in, each person it was too much trouble to help, pay attention to, or even see because he or she stood between my drugs of choice and me, was another tear in the fabric of my soul. Each time I didn't show up for life, until in the end I *couldn't* show up for life, was another step toward what would have been my eventual spiritual (and physical) destruction.

However, the soul is an exceptionally resilient thing. Unlike the body, it can be brought back to life. The principles of surrender, hopefulness, honesty, acceptance, and so on, as suggested in *The Soul Workout*, will affect you spiritually, but also physically, mentally, and emotionally. Following the suggestions in this book will help you build your character as well as your spiritual fitness.

The connection between small, everyday acts of kindness and spiritual growth is not unique to recovery. Many religions instruct believers to perform good deeds in order to express the world of the spirit through actions in the physical world. My childhood religion taught me about "The Corporal Works of Mercy." These included:

1. Feed the hungry.

2. Give drink to the thirsty.

3. Clothe the naked.

4. Shelter the homeless.

5. Visit the sick.

6. Visit those in prison.

7. Bury the dead.

Those instructions are specific, but how many of us, in everyday life, have the opportunity to visit prisoners or clothe the naked? Not many. What we can do, however, is break these instructions down into small, elemental parts. We can practice everyday acts of loving kindness. We can do *The Soul Workout*.

When I entered recovery, my spiritual vital signs were thready and almost indiscernible. Today, I exercise my soul through the practice of the Twelve Steps; through sponsorship, service, reading, and meeting attendance; and by the constant attempt to improve my "conscious contact" with God, as I understand God.

I do this in the prescribed ways, through prayer and meditation; however, for this addict, prayer and meditation occupy a discrete and often time-limited portion of every day. Life calls me out to live—to work, eat, sleep, love, and play. When I'm not in active prayer or meditation, I perform the actions of *The Soul Workout* with mindfulness that this is how I build my spiritual armor.

This book includes the small, easy-to-practice works of soul-building kindness and humanity I learned from my friends and teachers in recovery, as well as narratives detailing my transformation from a state of spiritual sickness to spiritual health.

The principles discussed in this book are those at work in the Twelve Steps of recovery. Those I write about are not the only ones there are; they are the ones I have recognized and attempted to develop within myself or live in since I reentered recovery in the mid-2000s. No step calls on or builds only one spiritual quality. Each quality is colored with and by the others, but all are necessary to build character, to strengthen spirituality, and to help you grow as a spiritual being.

By building spiritual practices into my everyday life, I began to rebuild my soul by "walking the talk," every day. You do not need to be a member of a twelve-step fellowship to benefit from this book. You do not need to be religious, either. I'm not. Anyone who wants to enrich his or her spiritual life and who is willing to do a few simple actions and think a few different thoughts can reap the rewards of *The Soul Workout.*

Be where you say you will be
when you say you will be there.

Practice saying, "Of course, I could be wrong."

Even when it doesn't seem to be working,
as long as you truly believe your
course of action is the right one, **don't give up.**
Results sometimes come in increments,
slowly, or not at all. Remember that you are
in the footwork business and your
Higher Power is in the results business.

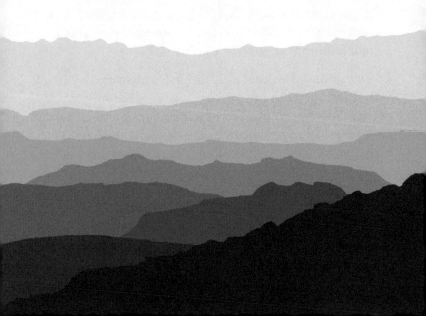

A WORD ABOUT SPIRITUALITY
(NOT RELIGION)

Finding a God of My Own Understanding

I entered Catholic school in the late 1950s when attending Catholic school still meant corporal punishment meted out by the overworked, overwhelmed, sometimes neurotic, sometimes kindhearted, sometimes vicious, sometimes sweet, often frustrated, usually angry, always orthodox creatures known to popular culture (and even to non-Catholics) as "the nuns."

The nuns ruled our lives inside the classroom and out. Even at home, our parents were subjected to "Sister says," especially whenever they looked like they were about to do something about which "Sister" had expressed disapproval. We girls were supposed to wear handkerchiefs pinned to the bodices of our dresses (never, *ever* trousers, not even during a New York City blizzard); I never remembered to wear mine. We were supposed to complete and turn in our homework. I didn't turn in my very first homework assignment. When I told my father, who was an alcoholic, that I was supposed to write out my spelling words five times each, he tore off a corner of a brown paper grocery bag, supervised as I wrote the words, and then said, "Good," before throwing the paper away. Try telling Sister Lurana that "I really *did* do my homework," when you don't have it written down in your brand-new, uncracked, black-and-white marble composition notebook like everybody else—even Richard Conboy, the "bad" kid from the broken home. I was not off to a good start in Nun World.

The nuns instructed us each to bring a quarter in a pink envelope once a week for our tuition and to have some additional small change every day so we could buy a piece of candy from a tin held by one of the favored "monitors." The proceeds went to "the missions" to buy a "black baby." I often wondered how my seatmate, Frank Bilberry—who, at that time, was the blackest person I'd ever seen and whose dark-as-midnight skin fascinated this pale-as-milk little Scottish-American girl—felt about that. We were shamed when we didn't have either the pink envelope or the so-called mission money.

With such qualities as the ability to instill an almost unnaturally keen understanding of English grammar into indifferent students and with a superhuman ability to diagram sentences, as well as an enthusiastic embrace of physical punishment as a pedagogical technique, the nuns had accepted the task of teaching Catholic theology to a sixty-member class of children of wildly disparate backgrounds, intelligences, and maturity levels. To do this they used the *Baltimore Catechism*, a teaching guide that, as I recall, consisted of a series of questions and answers that covered just about any aspect of Roman Catholic theology. The technique was breathtakingly simple; we memorized the questions and their answers alike, so when asked a question in class, we could parrot back the proper answer. I can still recall some from memory:

Q. Who is God?

A. God is the maker of heaven and earth, and of all things, visible and invisible. (The part about the "invisible things" always scared me.)

Q. What is man?

A. Man is a creature composed of body and soul and made in the image and likeness of God.

Q. Why did God make you?

A. God made me to know Him, love Him, and serve Him in this world and be happy with Him forever in the next.

And so on.

For some children, this method of indoctrination—lockstep reductionism and rigid control of everything inside the classroom and out, from the cleanliness of one's skin, clothing, and fingernails, to the movies one might and might not see with one's parents, to forced participation in almost-constant religious "processions," novenas, and children's masses, impersonally administered humiliations, unpredictably dispensed physical abuse, and the recitation of "horror stories" starring God's All-Stars, the martyrs—might have led to true spirituality and a love of God, although it was hard for me to see how. For others, it seemed to make no impression either way. Still others may have been irrevocably turned off to any idea of God, faith, or spirituality. For me, piled on top of the distorted ideas about God I was receiving at home from my well-intentioned mother, it created fear and anxiety, guilt and shame, a longing to know this God character, and a terrible fear of Him that existed simultaneously in my six-year-old heart and that lasted for most of my life.

During second grade, much classroom time was spent in preparing us for receiving our First Holy Communion; however, that couldn't occur until we'd all made our First Confessions. We were told that we needed to rid our young souls of all the sins we had committed during our first years of life in order to be proper receptacles for God's love, and, of course, to escape "the pains of hell," which were described to us in exquisite detail.

Trying to explain "sin" and "repentance" to six- and seven-year-olds couldn't have been easy. So if the nuns reverted to odd analogies, who can blame them? However, because of my early religious instruction, for many years I imagined my soul as being like nothing so much as a small dish towel, floating around inside my body—white, with fringed ends. That is, it was white until I committed a sin. Then my little dish towel got stained. Sometimes it got very badly stained, but even so, there was a miraculous washday solution to the problem of sin-soiled souls: the Sacrament of Confession, which had its own terrors, but at least held the promise of salvation and relief from pain.

During and after Catholic school, I would stray from and return to my religious roots repeatedly, especially during the years of my active addiction. I never grasped the reality of my spiritual nature until I entered recovery for what I hope is the last time. I know today that my soul is nothing like a little dirty dish towel.

My recovery fellowship has become my "religion," if by religion we can agree on a definition that includes a way of life and a set of principles, as well as a transcendent belief in a power greater than me.

In twelve-step recovery I've found my soul and a relationship with God as I understand Him today, which I see is not so far removed from the God who made me to "know Him, love Him, and serve Him," at least until my job in this world is done.

THE SOUL WORKOUT

**Pray, even though
you don't believe,**
and take actions you
don't think will work.

Look at others who are walking
on a spiritual path and **believe
that you, too, can follow.**

**Be aware of the
small miracles in your life.**

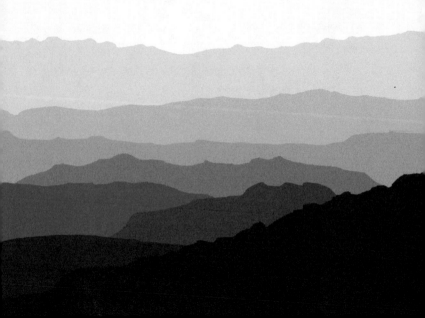

HONESTY

Looking at the Truth of My Life

I have been a liar all my life. When I was three or four, my mother sent me to our room—we shared one, along with my father and brother, until I was almost eight— with a whack on the backside for some transgression. Today I don't even remember what it was. What I do remember is that once over the threshold, I grabbed and started to swing the bedroom door, to slam it with all my three- or four-year-old anger and might, and as I did so, stuck my tongue out at my mother as vehemently as I could. What I had failed to take into account was that on the back of the door that I was slamming was a mirror. My parents' dresser, with its own mirrored top, stood against the opposite wall. My mother could clearly see me. I was busted by my own reflection. Fitting, wouldn't you say?

When my mother burst into the room seconds after the door slammed to confront me for my insolence, I compounded the felony by saying, with as much false innocence as I could muster (which was a lot, even back then), "I wasn't sticking my tongue out at you, Mummy! I was sticking it out at the devil! He's the one who made me be bad!" I admit, it's pathetic, but I was only three or four years old. The spanking that then commenced was much worse than the original whack that had sent me to my room. Isn't it interesting that my tongue got me into trouble—as it would continue to do for so many more years?

Whether or not I received spankings, I continued to lie. I lied to my mother, my father, my siblings, my teachers, my employers, my lovers, my husbands, and my friends. Why tell the uncomfortable truth when they won't understand it anyway? A lie is really just a timesaving device, and if it makes me look better than the truth would, so much the better. If it prevents me from laying out cash, better yet. If it gets me whatever I want and helps me avoid some unpleasant reality, that's best of all. At least that's what I used to think.

I lied myself right up to the brink of death and into recovery; even then, in the beginning, I lied to myself about why I was there. Now, a half-century after that tongue-poking incident, I'm finally learning how to be honest. And not just with my words.

I am a recovering member of a twelve-step fellowship; I do what I say I will do when I say I will do it, and I don't say things that aren't really so. And that's how my soul grows.

THE SOUL WORKOUT

If you let your child answer the phone, **please don't ever tell them to tell the caller you're not there.** It confuses and upsets them, and it teaches them that it's okay to lie.

When you don't know something, just say so. The amount of trouble this can save is amazing.

Have cash-register honesty. If they overcharged you a dollar, you would let them know. Let them know when they undercharge you a dollar, too.

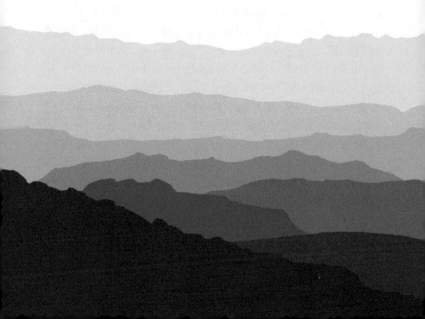

HOPE

Keeping My Chin Up

When I was about six years old, my father got a Bell & Howell black-and-white home-movie camera. Because of the technology of that time, the first movie he made was silent. It shows my mother, my younger brother, and me walking along a sunny sidewalk alongside a chain-link fence. On the other side of the fence, in a stranger's yard, was a swing set.

We lived in an apartment; we had no yard and no swing set, so this fenced-in plaything was tempting. On the movie screen, I see me holding my mother's hand like the good little girl I was always trying to pass myself off as—if not actually trying to be. I see my little brother lunging for that fence, and I note that I'm being edged out of the frame. My dad keeps the focus on Dougal, not quite four years old and already a devil, as he seeks to tear himself out of my mother's grip to climb the fence. The toes of his sneakers are just able to fit into the diamond-shaped interstices of the wire mesh. A struggle ensues, then the frame goes upside down and black as my father loses control of the camera, presumably to intervene and get Dougal back onto the sidewalk side of the fence. Then, when the film resumes, the focus is still on Dougal, swinging away and pumping his legs for all he's worth, having won another battle with my mother, and evidently with laws ranging from those of gravity to those regarding private property. He's smiling, and I'm nowhere in sight. I had always hoped to see myself in those old home movies, but somehow I never made the final cut.

All the old home movies are like this. In one reel, taken at Edinburgh Castle on our first trip back to Scotland as a family, I noticed my father was filming me. I hoped to do something entertaining enough to merit inclusion in the finished home movie, so I began dancing a childish, improvised "highland fling," which lasted scant seconds before I must have been yelled at to "quit it!" My smile disappears in an eye blink. My arms fall to my sides and my feet stop moving. Then I slink out of camera range and finally hide behind my mother. Onscreen, my disappointment and dashed hope are visible, almost palpable. I'm surprised my parents kept this reel, much less showed it. Hope disappointed is a heartbreaking thing to see on a child's face.

Over and over again throughout my childhood, I got the message that I needed to quit it and to shut up, NOW, when what I was hoping for was someone to listen to me, to look at me, to *see* me, and maybe even to appreciate me. I was a slow learner, though, because I kept on hoping the result would be different one day. I kept trying to stand up, no matter how many times I got hammered down. And I always got hammered down. Even today, the vision of hope disappointed on another person's face, especially a child's, can make me sob like nothing else.

I saw a movie once that was a highly fictionalized account of a man incarcerated in a maximum-security prison where a sadistic warden brutalizes him into murderous insanity. The maximum time an inmate was legally permitted to be held in "the hole" (solitary confinement) was seventeen days; however, this man spent three years there, stripped, bleeding, freezing, and beaten with clockwork regularity. The entire movie was brutal, but the scene that destroyed me emotionally was the one in which a cruel jailer opens the cell door, allowing the man to think he's finally going to get back into the general population after months in the hole.

The man's ruined, beaten face expresses pure, unbelieving joy, and you can see hope welling up in him—the hoping-against-all-hope he allows himself to feel, the hope that he will be able to feel sunlight on his face, experience human contact, and see sights other than those of the inky-dark hole for the first time in God-knows-how-long. Then, after only a half hour of freedom, he is thrown back into his solitary cell. All his hopes of freedom are crushed. With an animal howl, his transformation from man to murderous beast is almost complete; however, beasts do not hope. Only humans do or need to. That scene resonated with me, gave me nightmares, made me weep, and had me talking to my therapist for many sessions.

When my childhood hopes were crushed, my self-acceptance was crushed, too. I must have been hardheaded or a cockeyed optimist to allow myself to hope for recognition that was never going to occur. I eventually got the message that I was unacceptable. When self-acceptance goes, acceptance of others is almost impossible to achieve. Trust goes along with all of these things as well. How can you trust when your hopes are constantly dashed? How can you be optimistic when experience tells you that you will never achieve that thing you want so much? Yet hope, optimism, trust, acceptance, and self-acceptance are all so necessary to live a life of recovery. Without them, it's almost impossible to work and embrace the steps.

The poet Emily Dickinson called hope "the thing with feathers / that perches in the soul." Hope—the most necessary and most delicate and easily crushed emotion—is, paradoxically, the most resilient of spiritual qualities. When the mythic Pandora opened the box that let out all the evils into the world, one little speck of something very important remained at the bottom; that thing was hope. We need hope to counteract the many "evils" with which our lives are sometimes filled. I needed hope to move forward into recovery, hope that I could live as I saw others in recovery living, "happy, joyous, and free." Being desperate enough to hope once more, and trusting in the process, carried me through those early days and sustains me now as I work through the steps and try to practice the principles of twelve-step recovery in all I do.

Hope is a tender thing. Try to nurture it in others. They need it. And try to find it in yourself; you need it, too.

THE SOUL WORKOUT

When someone tells you what they're
hopeful about, like getting that
new job they just interviewed for,
**don't point out all the practical reasons
it won't happen.** Rather, wish them well.

Saying "better luck next time" builds hope.
Saying "I told you so" kills it.

Support "hopeless" causes—
e.g., prison reform, the elimination of land mines,
spay/neuter programs at local animal shelters.
You may never achieve total success, but you can
hope that you will make a difference.

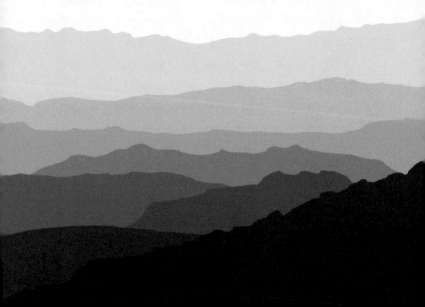

FAITH

Trusting in the Process

When I entered recovery, I needed *a lot:* a man, a car, a new job, money, dental work, etc., etc. The people in the rooms listened to me recount my problems and my woes. They smiled. They hugged me. They nodded. They said, "Work the steps."

"Maybe you didn't hear me," I tried to say. "How will working these stupid steps give me what I need?"

They smiled and said, "Work the steps."

So, I worked the steps.

I was desperate enough and broken enough to make a decision, as Step Three instructs, to trust in a power greater than myself and to trust that if I did as I saw others in recovery do—attend meetings, perform service work, and work the steps—things would work out for me, just as they promised. And that's what started to happen. Yes, I got a new car, a new job, and the needed dental work. What I didn't realize at the time, but know now, was that they were only the material signs that told me, "Help is on the way." The money? Well, this is about money. And trust… and faith.

Now that I've got some recovery time under my belt, now that the "gift of despair" is not so raw in me, sometimes I forget the magic found in the steps. I forget that when I began to follow the instructions outlined in the steps, even though not a single step says, "Stop engaging in your addiction," that's exactly what happened. Not only that; for the most part, I stopped wanting to. I certainly stopped being obsessed by it. When I worked the steps I didn't quite understand but worked them anyway, I discovered that I would receive a solution, not only to the problem of my addiction, but to the other problems in my life as well.

Like most people when they come into recovery, I owed money. A lot of money. Some of it to people who can put you in jail if you don't pay the money back. I took loans, I made arrangements, I paid off most of my creditors, and then I started paying back the loans. I made the best terms I could with some of my creditors, and some of those "best terms" were not too advantageous for me. Especially when I lost a long-standing freelancing gig and my rent-paying son moved out and I had to have a writing deadline pushed back that gave me more time to finish a manuscript, but delayed the date when I'd receive the second half of a much-needed advance.

One morning during this time, I contemplated calling the office of a law firm with which I had made payment arrangements, and to which I owed a monthly payment that was due that day. The idea of having to make that payment had been gnawing at the back of my mind like a rat. Delivering a check to them would deplete my account severely. It was only three days after payday, and paying what I owed would leave me less than four hundred dollars to live on for almost two weeks. "I should probably call them and see if they'll let me pay them two weeks from now, when I get my next paycheck," I told myself. I felt proud. Yes, I'd be honest and come clean with them. That sounded like "good program." I'd tell them I just didn't have the cash on hand to pay them on our agreed-upon due date; surely they'd understand. The problem with that was that I *did* have the cash on hand. I just didn't have much more than that. I just didn't have as much as I wanted. And I knew it.

However, I realized I had to be honest—I did have enough money to pay what I owed. I just didn't have enough to do that and buy Starbucks every day for the next two weeks. And cigarettes. And cute shoes. And go to the movies. No, I knew I had to pay what I'd said I would when I would, and I had to have faith that by acting with integrity and doing what I had promised to do, everything (including me) would be okay, just like when I first got into recovery. Working the steps and living according to spiritual principles seems to solve all my other problems.

Although I had a twinge of mistrustful panic, I went ahead and paid the full monthly payment that day. It was the arrangement I had worked out with the law firm. Even though cheese is four dollars a pound these days, gas is more than two dollars a gallon again, and the power company just filed another rate increase, I know I can live on less than four hundred dollars for two weeks. After all, some working people are raising families on less. My Higher Power has never let me down when I trusted and relied on Him and did what I knew was the next right thing. I decided I would not only have faith, I would act on faith.

When I sent off the check, the rat stopped gnawing at my brain and my anxiety abated. I had paid what I owed. I had faith that my Higher Power would provide for my needs for the next two weeks. And that's exactly what happened. Not only that, but the law firm arranged for me to meet with the creditor on whose behalf they were working, and as a result of honestly explaining my own part in the problem to that injured party, I received forgiveness, not just of the bulk of my debt to them, but of so much more. I received a measure of relief. This experience taught me a valuable lesson about honesty and trust in my Higher Power.

The Torah tells the story of Abraham, the patriarch of Israel, as an example of a life lived in absolute trust of a Higher Power. One day Yahweh told Abraham to sacrifice his only son, for whose birth Abraham had waited many long, childless years, and Abraham obeyed, taking the boy high up to the mountaintop where the two usually sacrificed sheep and lambs. The boy, Isaac, had no idea what was about to happen to him, but trusted his father, and carried the wood intended for his own pyre, unaware of what the wood would be used for. He even asked, "Father, what are we going to sacrifice?" when he noted they had brought no sacrificial animal with them. Abraham had no answer for his son. The two kept climbing up to the summit, which was the place of sacrifice. Abraham had faith in Yahweh's direction; he would obey, although his heart was sick with pain and the enormity of what he was about to do.

I've always been greatly moved by the faith of Abraham, and yet I've always thought Isaac's faith was greater. After all, in the tale, Abraham actually had been instructed by Yahweh, with whom he conversed freely. He had experienced the blessings Yahweh showered on him when he trusted. But Isaac hadn't. Yet he did as his father said, even though it made no sense to him, even though his father was not an omnipotent super-being. Isaac trusted his father absolutely.

Of course, you know how the story ended. An angel was sent to stop the sacrifice, and a ram miraculously appeared to take Isaac's place. Happy ending.

I want to have the faith of Isaac and to believe that my Higher Power will never ask more of me than I can give. I want to grow in trust and trustworthiness, as well. That's how I grow my soul.

THE SOUL WORKOUT

Let someone else drive. You may very well be the better driver, and you may very well know the way, but once in a while you need to experience having faith in others.

In situations where you really want a specific outcome and are tempted to manipulate or try to control people or things to get your desired result, just be aware that you are doing this and let go of it. **Trust the process.**

Have faith that no matter what happens, you will be okay. You may not get exactly what you want, but perhaps, to your surprise, you may get what you need.

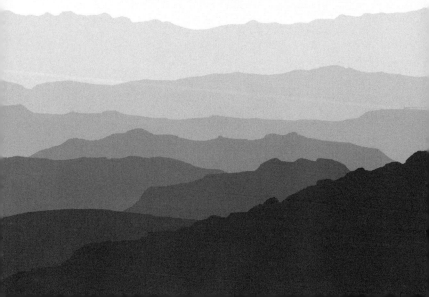

AWARENESS

Waking Up

I've heard people say in meetings that twelve-step recovery would be so great if "they didn't mess it up with that spiritual part." Spiritual *part*? I hate to break it to them, but there is no spiritual *part.* It's a *spiritual program.*

There is no way to break out the spiritual aspect of twelve-step recovery from the physical, mental, and emotional aspects, any more than there is a way to take the soul out of a person and have him or her live. We've all heard rumors of "zombies," but they are the stuff of horror and fantasy fiction.

Granted, many come to recovery "on the outs" with spirituality. Even though they are free to form their own conception of a Higher Power, they remain suspicious. "They say Higher Power, but I know they mean GOD" is their attitude. For many who have bottomed out, it seems that God has been silent, absent, or just plain cruel. How else to explain all the things that have happened to us? How else to explain tsunamis, stillbirths, and war?

Others have no trouble believing in a Higher Power; however, they believe he/she/it is responsible for all the bad things, like "giving" you cancer or punishing you for enjoying sex by "giving" you an STD. They desire no contact with such a power. Some have had terrible, fear-inducing "religious" upbringings. They fear and hate the very notion of God. And others look at all the inconsistencies religion seems to require they believe, such as the notion that while God created the world and everyone in it, he/she/it created some people with a nature that he (or she, or it) hates. Still others have come to a comfortable understanding that they do not and will not believe in a Higher Power of any kind. They may have faith in the spirit of humanity itself or in the power of nature, but they see no higher intelligence at work and feel no need to believe in one. The idea of God just does not ping on some people's radar. Whatever the reason, many people want no part of spirituality, which is most emphatically *not* religion or even a Higher Power of their own understanding.

In my life, I have passed through phases—from deeply held religious beliefs that never helped me resist my addiction or the behavior that stemmed from it, through atheism (all the atheists I knew were tough and cool, and since I was weak and nerdy, that seemed like a position I wanted to try on for myself), to an uncomfortable agnosticism, which is fine for some people, but to me it was finally just inauthentic and uncomfortable fence-straddling, because I inwardly longed for a connection with God. To say I was confused and had decided to have no part of spirituality when I entered recovery would be an understatement.

I was able to put aside the preconceived notions and the prejudices I had toward God or spirituality or even religion in order to "try" twelve-step recovery.

Whether you are in a recovery program or not, if you are seeking spiritual connectedness, you can also put aside your preconceived notions and try to remain aware that there just might be a Higher Power, a spirit that moves in you, me, and everyone. You might begin to see that Higher Power at work in your life, as I began to do, and still do today. As my friend Rupert says, he began to realize his Higher Power was working in his life after he stopped dismissing things as "just coincidences" and began looking for his Higher Power's will for him in events and people in his life. A Higher Power doesn't have to go by the name of "God." It may come in ways you don't expect, but it is more likely to come if you practice awareness.

Each morning at my home group, the secretary hands a copy of our basic recovery book to a member at random to select a reading, then share on it, and then pass to another member. Recently, one morning, the book was handed to me. A moment later, a very young man sat down at my table. He had nine days in recovery and was still vibrating, yet was looking for a loophole.

"Can I ask you a question?" he asked as he looked at me. I admit that I was annoyed. I had been leafing through the book, looking for a passage to read aloud that would give me the opportunity to be witty, wise, and moving, and possibly even launch a laugh or two. In other words, I was searching for a reading that would make me sound good and that would make the other group members like me more. "Sure,"

I said, unenthusiastically. All right, I was more than unenthusiastic; I was a touch peevish. Actually, it wouldn't be wrong to say I was condescending.

He pointed to a sentence. "This says, 'We have recovered,'" he complained. "But people in the program say we never really recover. That's inconsistent! Which is it?" Now, my Higher Power speaks to me in many ways—through you, through other people, and sometimes through inanimate objects. When I turn on the ignition in my car and the display reads "Perform Service," I think that's my HP talking to me, too. This time, HP spoke to me the way He sometimes does, in my head, right in back of my left ear. "Read the passage the kid is asking about" was the message I heard. So I did.

I read it, and I shared something, and then I called on another member to share, which is the way my home group runs. That member shared, and called on another, who called on another, and forty-five minutes later, as the meeting ended, the kid turned to me and smiled. "I get it," he said, and hugged me. "Thanks." Wow. I had watched the spirit of my Higher Power move around the room that morning like the beach ball at a Grateful Dead concert. It bounced from the secretary to me, to the kid, to each group member who shared, and then bounced right back to that young man who had nine days.

I try to remain aware of my Higher Power today, making certain assumptions, of course:

* ✴ I assume He exists;

* ✴ I assume He is crazy about me; and

* ✴ I assume He will speak to me in many ways if I remain attentive, conscious, and aware of His presence.

A speaker at a meeting I attended once talked about how important it is in recovery to be aware of the newcomer in his or her first thirty days—to encourage him or her and offer support. He went on to say that it's even more important to be aware of the person who may be in his or her last thirty days, who may be teetering on the brink of a relapse. That person needs our support and encouragement just as much as, if not more than, the newcomer. If we do not remain aware of ourselves and especially of the people around us, we might miss the opportunity to help save someone's life.

This applies to every one of us, not just those in recovery. Developing awareness of yourself, of your Higher Power, and of the people in your world will allow you to seize opportunities to build your soul that you would otherwise miss.

Be conscious of the feelings of others.
If someone near you is crying or is clearly upset,
don't look away. Look at him or her, and
ask if you can help. All he or she can say is no,
but your simple offer may make all the
difference in the world to that person.

Drive consciously and with kindness.
Remember that red means "stop"
and green means "go." Yellow does
not mean "go very fast."

Listen to understand, not just to respond.
If, in a conversation, while the other person is
talking you are busy formulating your reply,
you are not hearing anything he or she is saying
and you are treating that person as "less than,"
as in less than or less important than you.
This is disrespectful.

LOVE

Embracing a Power Greater than Me

My friend Eddie talks about his sponsor, Dave, a lot. Dave is a natural wit, a homegrown philosopher, and a madman. He's also a great example of recovery in action. Eddie is a member of my home group, and so I often get the benefit of Dave's wisdom when Eddie shares a "Dave story." One day, during the "open discussion" portion of our home group meeting, Eddie shared a story about a time, early in his recovery, when he was wallowing in self-pity and giving Dave an earful. Like any good sponsor, Dave listened for about a minute to Eddie's tale of woe and then stopped him in mid-wallow.

Like most Eddie-and-Dave stories, this one took place in Dave's car. That's where a lot of early recovery work happens, as sponsors with cars drive newcomers without cars to meetings. Eddie had no car of his own back then—no car, no house, no family, no job. He just had Dave and "the gift of desperation," which had led Eddie, as it leads so many of us, into recovery.

Driving down Las Vegas Boulevard one day, Dave and Eddie passed several homeless men holding cardboard signs, the same kinds of signs with the same pleas that homeless people carry in cities all over the world.

"Will work for food."

"Why lie? I need a beer."

"Homeless. Hungry. Please help."

"Disabled Vet."

As Dave and Eddie waited for a light to change, they noted that although there were at least fifty drivers idling at the four corners of the intersection, no one was opening a window to give money to the homeless guys. Dave took a drag on his cigarette, while Eddie took a break from his whining. "They need better signs," Dave said and smiled. Eddie just looked at him.

"If I were homeless," Dave said, gazing past Eddie to the panhandler approaching their car, "I know *exactly* what kind of sign I'd have." Eddie continued to watch him, waiting. This sounded like advice that might come in handy someday. The light changed, and they began to move, but not before Dave had handed some coins through the window and received a "God bless, man" in return.

"My sign wouldn't ask for money," Dave continued. "My sign would just say, **'Look what they've done to me!'** And I'd make a fortune from guys like you." And girls like me, because I would definitely give money to a guy with a sign like that, thinking, "Yeah! They're always trying to do things to *me*, too! Here you go!"

As Eddie tells the story, he was both puzzled and slightly offended.

"Whattaya mean, guys like *me*?" he asked Dave.

"Guys like you are guys who think someone else is to blame for what's wrong with their lives. You think you have low self-esteem, but what you really have is high self-pity. And it's gonna kill you if you don't get out of yourself and start thinking about others."

"Guys like Eddie…." Guys so full of self-pity and a conviction that their problems are not of their own making. I can relate. Simply substitute "girls" for "guys" and you're talking about me.

So what's a girl to do? And what does this have to do with love?

Quite a lot, actually.

Selfishness, self-pity, and self-centeredness all separate me from you, prevent me from seeing you as a fully formed human being with needs that I can actually help meet, once I stop trying so desperately to fulfill my own needs on my own. And, paradoxically, it's in trying to meet your needs to whatever degree I can that I am taken out of myself enough to let love in—love of my fellow human beings and love of life. Nothing I can try to grab, eat, drink, acquire, steal, ingest, manipulate, or use for myself can fill me up the way love for another human being can. Nothing can change me or build my soul the way love can. I needed to change. I was on a fast track to hell. My life now affords glimpses of heaven, which is where love lives.

But back to Dave and Eddie. I'm like most people who have never "lived outdoors," which is how some of my formerly homeless friends somewhat jokingly describe life on the street. Like most ordinary people, I find the homeless frightening. Their visual aspect and inadequate access to hygienic measures make them seem less than human and more like some grotesque and monstrous alien life-forms. It's hard to remember that there is a human being under there. Hard to remember what my mother used to say whenever she'd give money to a panhandler: "That was somebody's baby once."

After spending a couple of years in meetings in a dingy church basement, under flickering fluorescent lights, drinking bad coffee, sitting on a rickety chair next to guys who stank, and seeing the light come back on in their eyes, I've come to know that there really is a human being under a homeless person's appearance, and with a little kindness, that human being can emerge and begin to live a life of recovery. It can start with a simple, conscious gesture of love. The healing power of love is certainly a power greater than me.

Should I ever need a sign, I know what it will say: **"This Could Be YOU."** If I always remember this could be ME, I will be a long way toward remembering to treat others with compassion, tolerance, and love.

I've learned in recovery that there are times it's perfectly okay to give money to a homeless man or woman, but that when I do, I must make every effort to look into their eyes, to say something kind, and to smile at them. When I place coins into their hands, I make sure the skin of my hand touches theirs for a moment. I try not to just look at them, but to look into them, to see the spirit of God that I believe resides in us all. When they thank me, I try to remember to say, "Thank YOU," before I drive away into my really quite beautiful life.

THE SOUL WORKOUT

Practice the "Golden Rule": Do unto others
as you would have others do unto you.

**Keep in mind that everyone is
deserving of love.** Give love unconditionally
and receive it in the same way.

Don't talk about how much you love your kids;
show it by spending time with them and,
of course, paying your child support.

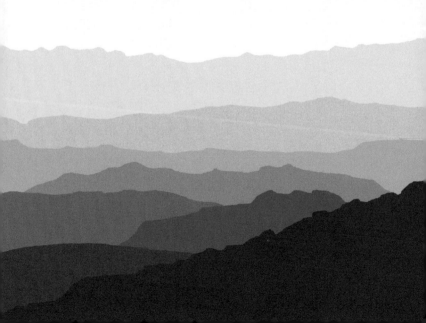

POWERLESSNESS

Accepting My Freedom to Be Me

I first entered recovery at the age of forty. My addiction, which began slowly in my late teens and grew during my twenties, had roared ferociously through my thirties, and by the week of my fortieth birthday it had reached previously unplumbed depths. I didn't, wouldn't, or couldn't see those depths for what they were—the depths of degradation. I thought I was having fun, and I felt that it was about time. At the age of forty, I was earning my own money and spending whatever wasn't "demanded" by my "selfish" spouse to contribute to the upkeep of our home and family on myself and my addiction. I thought I was expressing my freedom—the freedom to do, say, think, and especially, drink whatever I wanted and as much as I wanted. Anything that stood in the way of what I wanted was a grave impingement on what I saw as my freedom. The reality was that my addiction had me enslaved.

Like so many who first enter recovery, I was secretly terrified that something would prevent me from getting my next high, and terrified of losing my "freedom" to indulge in my disease. I did not know and would not have accepted, even if it had been pointed out to me, that my addiction was the master of my body and soul. It controlled my life and forced me into an isolation that kept me from being the wife, mother, employee, citizen, and person I now know I was dying to be. It twisted my thinking. Freedom? What kind of freedom was that?

Every aspect of my life, from the moment I came to in the morning until I passed out at night, I was under the thrall of my obsession. I was either working enough to earn the money to get loaded, getting loaded, or getting over getting loaded. I was bitter, angry, and belligerent or self-pitying and self-dramatizing, raging and pouting or maudlin and weepy or self-justifying and sneaky. I was never free to be me.

I had no intention of discovering a relationship with my Higher Power or even of stopping using forever. I didn't want to stop using; I only wanted to eliminate the consequences of my using. I wanted to wipe the look of disgust off my husband's face. I wanted to hang onto my job, my home, my freedom, and my kids. That was all. Little did I know how much more I would get someday. For me, recovery was to be punctuated by relapse, but I couldn't foresee that. I just wanted the pain to stop.

I entered outpatient rehab—four subway rides, two nights a week, two hours a night—for a year and a half. I went to my job as a book editor in Greenwich Village during the day. I continued writing children's books that continued to be published. I began attending twelve-step meetings at the instigation of my rehab counselor. "Why do I need to go to meetings?" I'd pout. "Because you can't stay in rehab forever," he'd answer.

I started going to meetings. In those days, in my neighborhood, the ratio of men to women at meetings was high, and I was told I needed to be sponsored by a woman, so I asked one of the few women I saw at meetings to sponsor me. She was pleasant and kind, had been in recovery much longer than I had, and had no more idea of how to sponsor me than I had of how to be sponsored. We talked about her son in prison, we talked about my job, we talked about New York news, but we never talked about what mattered. We never talked "program," we never read our fellowship's recovery book, and we never worked the Twelve Steps. I do not blame her; she just didn't know better.

The words "Higher Power" were mentioned in every meeting I attended, and I said the Serenity Prayer at the beginning of each meeting and the Lord's Prayer at the end. I affirmed that I did in fact believe in a Higher Power; however, in retrospect, I realize that my Higher Power at that time consisted of my husband and children. I now know that children grow up and husbands run away with women they meet while country-and-western dancing, but I didn't pick up my drug of choice. I had a dry kind of recovery. Physically, I was getting better, as was my life. I kept my job and prospered there. My husband was able to exhale, no longer afraid of what "fresh hell" I was getting him into whenever I was out of his sight. My children were growing into splendid young men. I wrote more books. I stayed in recovery, attended meetings, enjoyed the fellowship, and was free from the phenomenon of craving. That is, until after the you-know-what hit the fan.

By the time it did, my family and I had moved across country and were living well in a beautiful new home. We enjoyed living near my sister and her family in a much different part of the country where we could swim every day during the long, golden sunset in our own pool, where getting to work didn't involve buses and subways, and where the days were long and hot and exciting. It was also where my first husband met his second wife.

Before we made our big move from the East Coast, I had stopped going to meetings, thinking I could "handle" recovery on my own. I made the mistake too many in recovery make—I let myself believe that recovery was something like a degree program and that I could master and complete it like a skill or trade. Recovery had given me many gifts, including health, improved relationships, and financial security. I felt good. I "had it," or so I thought. I was still physically abstinent, but I had no program, no spirituality, and certainly no relationship with my Higher Power. I was in control. I was a relapse waiting to happen.

When my husband and I finally divorced, after twenty-six years of a turbulent and often distressing marriage,

I wasted no time finding and marrying husband number two. He was everything my first husband hadn't been. He was tough, he was macho, he was overtly sexy, he was funny as hell, he was smart, and he was in active addiction.

I fell in love with him like a dry tree in a lightning storm. I just caught fire and went up in a ball of flames. He loved me back, passionately, and he courted me so beautifully that I began to believe that I really *was* the most beautiful, the most intelligent, the sexiest, and the most desirable woman in the world; and oh, by the way, I was no longer an addict. I had just "overcorrected." Today I know better. I know that when a man starts worshipping at the church of St. Helen, Helen then starts to believe she is God. A dangerous delusion for this addict, because it leads me to think I'm my own Higher Power.

But I didn't know that then, so I took what my "disease of perception" told me was a desirable course of action: I chose to pick up and started using my drug of choice. I relapsed and married my man and we had a great time, for a short while. Too short. By our third wedding anniversary, he had the first of his numerous hospitalizations with pancreatitis. The next two years of our lives together were a hell of hospitalizations, physical and moral disintegration, using, blackouts, mysterious injuries, surgeries, transfusions, illnesses, and finally, his death at the age of fifty-one.

He died in my arms in a pool of blood, and he died drunk. I got a lot of mileage out of his death. As the grieving widow, I had the world's best excuse to get loaded, I thought. I nearly followed him into the grave myself. I became a regular at local emergency rooms and detox facilities. My sons, two of whom were by this time grown and fathers themselves, would come to visit and leave quickly, shaking their heads and never quite trusting me around my grandchildren, who seemed to be arriving on the planet with increasing frequency. My job performance was a joke, and I was a fixture in the human resources department.

My appearance suffered. Far from the beautiful and sexy woman I was on my wedding day to my second husband, I now was a fat, bloated, creaking, red-faced wreck, much older than her years. I had developed eczema, a common and extremely unattractive ailment for addicts of my type. My blood pressure was so high I suffered frequent projectile nosebleeds. I needed a gastroenterologist on call. Every single morning for the last two years of my active addiction, I went through withdrawals. I had uncontrollable tremors, sweating, tachycardia, double vision, vomiting, dry heaving, and numbness in both hands, and was unable to make my legs work. Two months before I would eventually enter recovery again, I was released from my nearby hospital, holding in a shaking hand a paper confirming what I knew deep inside. I was dying from the disease of addiction.

So began my slow trudge back into the rooms of twelve-step recovery. My last hospitalization was in March 2007, and by May 10 of that year I was on the road back to a life in recovery. I got a sponsor who had a sponsor who had a sponsor. I got my old recovery book off the shelf, blew off the dust, and this time I read it. My sponsor wasted no time in guiding me through the steps. I got a home group and a service commitment. I made friends with the women in the program. All this happened much more slowly than it takes to write or read it, of course, but it happened. I jumped into recovery with both feet, and this time I actually worked the steps.

With Step One, I admitted I was powerless over my addiction. As time passed and I worked the program, I realized that this powerlessness extended to just about every area of my life. I am powerless over world events, over the weather, over my children's lives and those of their wives and my grandchildren. I am powerless over how other people perceive me and even over how they treat me.

This realization of powerlessness is in fact the foundation of my recovery. It keeps me far away from "slippery" persons, places, and things. It allows me to be responsible only for my own actions, but to be fully responsible for them. It permits me to let God be God. It lets me know that I'm neither the best person in the world nor the worst, and that I'm just as my Higher Power intended me to be, and that's enough.

I've learned that powerlessness is not helplessness. I am certainly not helpless. I've been given everything I need to make my way in this world. Today I use my intelligence, talents, and heart to work the steps, help others, and enjoy my beautiful, God-given life every day.

Accepting powerlessness is accepting freedom; it allows the weight of the world to fall from my shoulders. Accepting my powerlessness goes hand-in-hand with trusting my Higher Power to provide everything I need.

THE SOUL WORKOUT

When you leave the house without
your cell phone, **consider the possibility that
your Higher Power is holding it for you** so you
don't have to be stressed out by phone calls.
Unless you are waiting for a liver transplant,
there is probably no call so important that you
need to rush back and find your phone.

Fall in love.

Enjoy the ride; don't just
look forward to the destination.

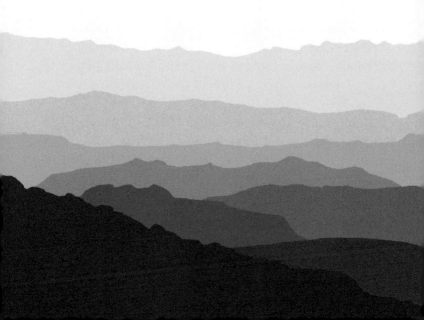

EXPECTATIONS KILL

Letting Go to Grow

I killed a pigeon one day, right after my second anniversary in recovery. It was completely unintentional. In fact, until it happened, I had been under the impression that it was impossible to kill a pigeon.

I grew up and, for many years, lived in New York City. Like every New Yorker, I know that a pigeon will always get out of the way of your car, no matter what. You cannot close the distance between yourself and a pigeon with a car. That's a fact. Yet, one bright May morning in Las Vegas, after saying my prayers and virtuously heading on my way to my home group meeting, I did that very thing.

It's not like I didn't see the pigeon. I saw him clearly as he stood in the middle of the street. He also seemed to see me. He was looking at me with his little pigeon eyes as I bore down on him slowly, expecting him to disappear for a second beneath the hood of my car, and then reappear a second later to my right or left, flapping his wings violently as he flew to safety. Except he didn't. And when he didn't, I had an "uh-oh" moment. Then, suddenly, the whole event took on a cartoonlike quality—for me, but not for the pigeon, I'm sure. There was a muted "whomp," then a grisly, grinding, bumping sensation as my front tire killed him and my rear tire crushed his corpse. I kept driving. Then, in the rearview mirror, there was the proof: a diffuse and dispersing cloud of gray and white feathers rose swirling from the pavement and eddied in the draft of my Jeep as I drove away from what had become the scene of minor carnage.

I winced and said a prayer, on the off chance that pigeons have souls. I said a prayer for me, too, asking my Higher Power what He was trying to teach me by putting a pigeon with a death wish in my path so soon after I'd celebrated a recovery milestone. And not only a recovery milestone. I realized that I was in love with the man I'd been seeing for the past month or so, embarking on the first romantic relationship I'd ever had that was free of the influence of my active addiction. Was the death of the pigeon an omen? What was my Higher Power telling me with this mysterious event? What could I learn from this? One of the first things my sponsor taught me in recovery, by her words and actions, is that when you start from the assumption that what *is* is God's will, then there's always something to learn. If I remain conscious, open-minded, and aware, it's always to my benefit.

One thing that occurred to me almost instantaneously was that the pigeon didn't behave the way I'd expected a pigeon to behave. Did I end his life because I'd acted on an expectation?

Expectations kill.

Think about the times your expectations have killed your enjoyment of a holiday, a family get-together, a new job, a new car, a new love. How disappointed and mystified were you when those expectations weren't met? How much more miserable was your misery because it contrasted so sharply with what you had expected? Rest assured, you are not alone. The same consumer magazines that are filled each autumn with articles exhorting you to have your "best holiday ever" are also filled with the dangers of letting your expectations get too high. It's maddening! "Have the Best Holiday Ever!" trumpet the headlines, but don't get too bummed when it's more Beverly Hillbillies than Beverly Hills. Yeah. Right. We all suffer, not so much from too-high expectations as from any expectations, period. Okay, then. What to do? It's not enough to let go of negative principles, which leave a vacuum when they go. This addict wants that vacuum to be filled with dangerous things. Letting go of expectations requires replacing them with the spiritual principles of openness, willingness, and faith.

Learning how to let go of expectations in recovery helped me embark on a remarkable love relationship when the right man appeared in my life after I'd almost resigned myself to remaining a lonely single widow forever. "Well," I'd tell myself unconvincingly, "I *had* two husbands, and they were good men. Maybe that's my quota." But the truth is that I was isolated and unfulfilled, and in my heart, I was longing to love again.

I actually didn't think I had expectations of my own when I began to look for a potential partner. I knew I really didn't have a "type" in mind (unless Sean Connery counts as a "type"). I knew I wanted someone smart and kind and who could make me laugh without taking his clothes off. When I whined about my loneliness, my sponsor suggested an age-old exercise: "Make a list of the qualities you want in a man and try to embody those qualities yourself. That's the kind of man you'll attract." It sounded strange, but then, so did many of the suggestions I received in early recovery. Those strange suggestions had worked in every other area of my life, so I figured, what did I have to lose?

I followed my sponsor's instructions and made a list, and because I'm a poet, it came out as a poem. When I started out, I could only think of the things I didn't want, and that's where I began.

MAN WANTED

I do not want to be a nurse,
I do not want to be a purse,
I do not want to squeeze your zits,
Just want a friend with benefits.

I do not want to trim your nails,
Do not want *you* to trim *my* sails,
I did not say you were a louse,
I just don't want you in my house!

"Can I wash your car for you?"
"I'd rather that you just washed *you*."

"Would you like it in the tub?"
"I'd rather have a nice foot rub.

"I wonder what you're like in bed?"
"I have a feeling *you're* half-dead."

"Does your mother bother you?
Forget it, I'm a mother, too."

"What do you want? I'm just a man!"
"And there's the problem, Stan or Dan."

I do not want a Stan or Dan or
Any other kind of man
To sofa-surf and watch TV,
That's just not fun, so leave me be!

I don't want someone else's gas,
Underneath my nose to pass,
When I'm all settled for the night,
Your "oven" needs a pilot light.

No golfer, dentist, private eye
For this position need apply,
No NASCAR Dad or CPA
You guys can all just go away.

No aging rock stars,
Businessmen,
Or guys who go to bed at ten,
(And really, who would go to bed
With a flaming dittohead?)

No racist,
Sexist,
Homophobe,
(I'd rather have an anal probe.)

A mountain climbing baby-boomer?
I'd rather a malignant tumor,

A tattoo-parlor devotee?
I'd wish he would just go away,

A healthy, hale US Marine?
(Don't think he'd fit into my scene.)

A redneck with a gun and rack?
(I think I'd have a heart attack.)

A hunter who can trap a bear?
Forget it, and get OFF my HAIR!

Do you like a dance with death?
A little hit of coke or meth?
A little snort, a little shot?
For you, I'm not so hot to trot.

After a month or two, I was finally ready to start thinking about what I *did* want.

MAN WANTED: PART *DEUX*

I hear it now; I know you're pissed,
Your manly hand balled in a fist,

You say the words
Men always say,
You speculate

I must be gay,
You fume and fret, your face turns blue,
But really, it's not me—it's YOU!

Yet if you have
These traits I've listed,
Prepare to get
A little twisted,
A little torn,
A little teased,
A little porn
A little pleased…

Please have two eyes, a nose, some teeth,
Have some on top *and* underneath,

It's okay if your pate's not hairy,
As long as what you've *got's* not scary.

And if you dance, that's better yet,
(And if you dip, you'll get me wet.)

If you don't have a car, okay,
But you *should* have a place to stay.

If you can make me laugh, get to it
Just don't take off your clothes to do it.

And if you can't "get with my friends"
Please know that here our friendship ends.

I hit "save" and prayed for my Higher Power to provide me with the man I just described. I didn't think I was asking for much—some hair, some teeth (even store-bought), his own place, and a personality. I didn't think that list contained unrealistic expectations. True, it was kind of vague, but at least it was something. When I shared the list with my sponsor, she revealed the kicker. "Now *you* try to be that person you wrote about. That's the sort of person you'll attract." Sponsors! I did what she suggested and started, tentatively, dating again.

When I first met Roger, I felt awkward and unsure of myself. Frankly, I was afraid. I had been a widow for almost four years and in recovery for almost two. My foundation in recovery was good; I was reasonably sure of that. I was attending meetings, I had service commitments, I read and reread recovery literature, I prayed and meditated, and I had worked the steps. Twice. I was ready for a new romance, of that I was certain. What I wasn't ready for was what it would be like to experience another human being in a romantic relationship without mood- or mind-altering substances and their concomitant behaviors as a lubricant. On those first few dinner, movie, and coffee dates, I felt anxious, self-conscious, and gauche. I expected I would feel the way I had when I started dating husband number one, at the age of fifteen, or husband number two, at age forty-five, filled with immediate desire and the sure knowledge that this was "the one." No wonder I couldn't feel any sparks. With those expectations, there wasn't room for a spark to ignite.

After about five weeks of spark-free dinner dates, I called my sponsor.

"I think I need to break up with Roger," I told her. "I'm not feeling anything. He's very nice, but I don't think there's any chemistry there. I mean, to me, a man is like a dress. If you buy a dress just because it's on sale or it's your size or it might be okay to wear to work, it's still gonna be hanging in the closet with the tags on it six months from now; and it's gonna hang in the closet 'til you send it to Goodwill. It doesn't become more attractive with time."

"Hm-hmm."

"So what is the best way to break up with him? I mean the most ethical way? Should I just let the whole thing die a natural death?"

Silence.

"Should I do it over the phone?"

More silence.

"Or should I send him an email?"

"You should pray to your Higher Power and follow your heart. You'll know what to do then."

Click. *Sponsors!*

I took my sponsor's advice and arranged to see a movie with Roger that weekend. Before I left the house on the prearranged evening, I sincerely asked my Higher Power to give me the gift of "no expectations" to help me allow the evening to wash over me, and to allow Roger just to be Roger, sparks or no sparks. I asked to be able to see Roger as he really was and to realize that he was not my ex-husband, or my late husband, or any other guy I'd ever met. I met him for our date that evening and what followed was remarkable, and full of the sparks I hadn't expected would turn up so long after a first meeting. My entire feeling toward him began to warm and change. To tell you the truth, it felt like there were sparks, after all.

When I look back at my expectations of my dating experience, I realize that if I had met the sort of man I fantasized about, I wouldn't be in a relationship right now. I'd most likely be licking my wounds and devouring cookie dough ice cream while listening to Gloria Gaynor CDs. The man my Higher Power had in store for me is not what I had expected, but much more. He is someone kind, funny, and smart, who is a good father and a good son, an amiable companion, a good-natured partner, and a generous lover who turned out to be crazy about me. If I hadn't asked my Higher Power for help in letting go of my expectations and living in acceptance, I would have missed out on this man, who has changed my life and brought me great fulfillment and true happiness.

Learning to live without expectations takes practice. Our brains have evolved to make use of our expectations as a survival skill. We expect that our days will unfold as they always have and the result is sometimes calm and a sense of security, but just as often a sense of boredom or dissatisfaction. We begin to crave excitement and to seek out the unexpected, only to be disappointed when it turns out to be unexpected in a way we're not really prepared for. We retreat into our familiar expectations. The cycle starts again. How do we strike a balance?

One way I've learned to do this is by maintaining conscious contact with my Higher Power, asking always for the strength to meet whatever He sends me, and the awareness that I am always in His care, no matter how scary or upsetting unexpected events in my life may become. Rereading that last sentence, I realize it contains a misstatement, "asking always." Truth is, I ask when I remember to ask. Sometimes I forget. But in recovery, I have discovered a fellowship of friends who always remind me of what I need to do, and sometimes they remind me to breathe and to ask God to show me what I need to see, letting go of expectations along the way.

Hold the door open for the person behind you, and don't get annoyed if he or she does not thank you. Don't do what I used to do and call out after the person in my most sarcastic voice, "You're welcome!" Be glad you were able to help.

Try new foods with an open mind.

If you're getting engaged or married or having a baby, don't use a gift registry. For your next birthday, **don't tell others what you want or what to get you,** even if they ask. Let people give you what they want to give you, and thank them for whatever they give.

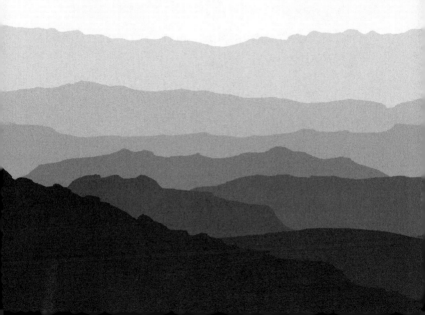

INTEGRITY

Taking Responsibility for My Actions

"Getting into a relationship in recovery is like putting fertilizer on your character defects." So says my beautiful redheaded friend Kitty. To which I can now say, "Amen."

I had been widowed for two years when I entered recovery. When I stopped using, I was a fat, bloated, coarsened wreck of a middle-aged woman, not likely to appeal to any partner (even by my own estimation), so following the time-tested recovery advice not to date for the first year was not very difficult. There wasn't exactly a line of men who wanted to get to know me. My dance card was blank. I was a mess. And that was just on the outside.

When I stopped putting substances into my body and I began recovering physically, mentally, emotionally, and spiritually, I uncovered a mass of feelings I'd been burying under my active addiction. I thought I had grieved my husband at the time of his death, when in fact I used his death to allow my disease to explode, until I nearly followed him into the grave. When I pulled myself out of the death spiral and staggered into the rooms of recovery, those buried feelings began to surface, which is an almost universal recovery experience. Although I was lonely and, as time passed, would become extremely frustrated, I was in no shape to either attract a potential partner or engage in a healthy relationship during my early recovery. I took my sponsor's advice and concentrated on working my program for my first year. However, when I was well into my second year and still had no romantic prospects, I began to lose heart.

"I'm just glad I never had to prostitute myself," I complained to my sponsor, "because evidently I can't even get a guy to date me for free!" Joyce would smile and shake her head and then tell me, with great confidence, that my Higher Power had someone in mind for me and that He was getting me ready for a real relationship. All I had to do was stay patient and continue to work the program of recovery. That is not an easy order for an addict, at least not easy for this one.

When I finally found myself in my first relationship in recovery, I had lots of good advice from my sponsor and program friends:

"Keep things in perspective."

"Just enjoy each other."

"Stay in the moment."

"One day at a time."

Now I can laugh at myself and the overconfidence I acted on in embarking on this affair.

Him: "I'll get emotionally attached."

Me: "Don't worry about it; I've got a program."

Yeah, right. My "perspective" went the way of all flesh, although thankfully my program didn't, and I fell for this delightful man, hard. I had all the symptoms:

* ❋ I couldn't eat.

* ❋ I couldn't sleep.

* ❋ I couldn't think of anything except him.

* ❋ I wanted to talk about him to everyone, including random strangers in line at the 7-11!

"Oh, wow! You like Slim Jims, too? My boyfriend likes Slim Jims!"

At this time, I had been working for about seven months at a new job. My boss, an understanding member of a twelve-step fellowship herself, was someone I could (and did) confide in about my new love. She was sympathetic; she was happy for me; she was another source of good advice. And she was concerned. With good reason. A good worker can become a bad one overnight, where love and addiction are concerned.

The first time Roger sent roses to the office, I was delighted. Every girl likes to get red roses, especially when they're delivered at work. I'm not so spiritually fit yet that I'm above enjoying a little jealousy on the faces of my female coworkers. When Roger showed up in the office parking lot one day at closing time, just because he couldn't wait until that night to see me, it was like injecting my ego with steroids. I began to believe that whatever pretty things he told me about my amazing and unique wonderfulness were objective truth, rather than recognizing them for the perfectly sincere and heartfelt, yet nevertheless almost universal, "sweet nothings" any man in love offers his woman.

After the roses and the after-work trysts, things went from great to even better in the bedroom, and from bad to worse everywhere else. I kept forgetting to eat. I began forfeiting sleep in favor of sex-and-talking-all-night, then smoked more cigarettes and drank more coffee during the day in an attempt to counteract the effects of sleep deprivation. As anyone who's tried this can attest, this still leaves one sleepy, but with the added annoyances of the jitters and a nicotine headache. My dog's walks became shorter and shorter. I made all my usual twelve-step meetings, but I began arriving late, and when the Serenity Prayer was recited, my thoughts were south of the equator, definitely not on my Higher Power.

At the office, things were even worse. My mind was completely preoccupied with thoughts of Roger— what we had said and done the previous night or where we would go and what we might do that weekend. My work output suffered at precisely the time my boss needed my help in order to meet our sales and marketing deadlines. I was about as useless as I'd been since the first week in the job, when I couldn't have been expected to be very productive. In effect, I was stealing from my employer. I was accepting a day's pay for sitting at my desk not doing a day's work. My boss had me in for "a talk."

Everything she said to me was perfectly true and just. I sat across the desk from her like a bobble-head doll, nodding in agreement. I was clocking in every morning and sitting in front of my keyboard all day, but my productive output was close to nil. My boss told me she was very concerned, pointed out the discrepancy between her and our employer's expectations and my actual "deliverables," and left me with the option to shape up. Fast.

The good thing about having a boss in recovery is that I can ask her advice. "What do you do when you're preoccupied and distracted and your mind wants to be anywhere but where you are?" I asked her. She told me that of course she had many concerns and issues, like everyone else—the economy, her health, her planned purchase of a home, dealing with financing, etc., etc…. "When my head starts spinning and I go off into thoughts of all these things that I'm concerned about," she said, "I imagine a red STOP sign. I see it and I tell myself to stop spinning off into these unproductive and anxiety-producing thoughts. It works for me. I don't know what might work for you, but I do know that when you clock in to this office, I need you to *be* in this office. Not off somewhere in your head with Roger." She smiled, but she was serious. She hugged me before I left her office, which was reassuring. I knew she was right.

Once back at my desk, the first thing I did was to print off a large image of a STOP sign, and place it above my monitor. I prayed to my Higher Power, "Dear God, remove these thoughts and feelings from me and direct my attention to what you would have me be." I had to repeat that prayer many times in the next day and a half, but eventually I was able to concentrate almost 100 percent on my work. I was able to "box up" my thoughts and feelings about my new love and realize I could always return to them later. I was able to obey the sign above my desk and STOP! As more days passed, I was able to be a productive and "present" employee once more.

I really was able to return to my thoughts and feelings about Roger and our relationship any time I wanted, which I realized needed to be after working hours.

Integrity means delivering what I say I will deliver. As an employee, I agree to perform certain tasks for a certain number of hours a day in exchange for a certain salary and benefits. When I am unproductive and "not present," I am actually stealing from my employer.

Today I am a member in good standing of a twelve-step program of recovery. I can take pride in doing what I say I will do when I say I will do it, in being where I say I will be when I say I will be there. I can hold up my end of a bargain. Sometimes I need a reminder, such as the one I got from my boss, but by using the tools of the program— prayer, meditation, sponsorship, and the principles of rigorous honesty and self-examination—I was able to return to productivity and be an honest employee again.

THE SOUL WORKOUT

Wash your hands after you
use the public restroom—
even if no one else is in there.

**Don't commit to anything
until you are sure you can do it,**
and then follow through with
your commitment.

Pay your taxes. Don't cheat.

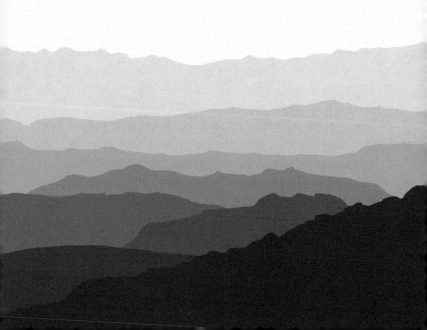

RESENTMENTS

Seeing My Part in Things

I never imagined I'd ever be a stepmother, but if I had thought about it, I wouldn't have wanted to be an "evil" one—although I do quite like the outfit Disney's animators created for Snow White's evil stepmother. After all, I already had mothered three sons and was busy as the hands-on grandmother of their five children by the time the possibility of becoming a stepmother arose in my life.

When I started dating after a couple of years in recovery, I told anyone who asked, "I'm through with production; I'm now in research and development." Then I found myself in a relationship with Roger and his teenaged son. It was not a Jerry Springer kind of relationship, just a human one.

I always had considered myself "good with kids," but the stepmother role is fraught with difficulties the mother role doesn't have to face. I knew how to be a mother, and in spite of everything, including my active addiction, I believe I was a good one. Not as good as I could have been, of course, but I'm satisfied that I was good enough. I wasn't in full-blown addiction for most of my sons' childhoods; I just wasn't ever completely "there" when they were young. But they've turned out to be terrific young men, so I guess I was "there" enough. My first husband, their father, Sal, gets a lot of the credit for the way they turned out.

Parenting with Sal was one of the few things we did well together or did together, period. We were like many couples in difficult marriages. Raising our children was one of the few areas in which we could feel and express spontaneous joy, work together toward a common goal, share common values, work as a team, and experience the same kind of love at roughly the same moment. It was one of the few areas in which we could enjoy our lives together. The children we had were, and still are, a source of love, strength, and satisfaction to me. Even through the worst of times, my sons and their love have always sustained me and brought me joy. One day in 1999 our family fell apart, and soon after that, my sons had a stepmother. I never thought they would one day have a stepmother or that I would one day have the chance to be one to another boy. My experience with that role was an extreme spiritual challenge at first.

In my "previous life," I assumed that by the simple virtue of our being their parents, my sons' father and I would always remain together, despite our unhappiness, and endure a quietly desperate marriage that would focus, in our old age, on our growing family of children, in-laws, grandchildren, and great-grandchildren. When our marriage did end—and it was a surprise to me when it did, mainly because I'd always assumed that if there were ever going to be any serious leaving, *I'd* be the one to do it, not him—this fantasy died, as well. Then, years later, in recovery, when I fell in love with a man who had a teenaged son, I had the opportunity to take on the "stepmother" role myself.

Any woman who dates a widower whose wife died when his son was under the age of ten will brush up against that boy's anger, resentment, grief, loneliness, puppy love, and growing pains. And puberty. And video games. And ninja moves. Because I prided myself on being "good with kids," I made assumptions that would be tested in my new role as Evan and I got to know each other.

One night very early in his father's and my relationship, I was in my car with Roger's son, Evan, running some errands. It seemed that the moment his seat belt was fastened he exploded into a diatribe worthy of a political news pundit in full campaign season, apropos of nothing I could see. I was truly puzzled and shocked. What possibly could have triggered this? Was it something I said? But I hadn't said anything. He began verbally unloading on me, raging on topics from the global to the particular, with the general theme being "my life sucks and it's someone else's fault. And my dad never lets me have any fun." Was there ever a teenage boy who didn't feel this way? I let Evan vent for a few minutes while my pulse hammered and I tried to figure out how to put a stop to the flow of (to me) shockingly venomous abuse this hitherto calm and polite young person was unleashing. The best I could finally come up with was a few mumbled, stammering bromides ending with, "Evan, I am probably the absolute worst person in the world for you to be having this conversation with."

There was a moment of thunderous silence; my grip on the steering wheel tightened and I braced myself. I was afraid he might just have been "reloading." But no, he seemed to have processed at least the last part of what I'd said. He took a beat. When he spoke again, I was treated to a disquisition on the merits of Dragonball Z vs. Grand Theft Auto, without a pause for breath for the rest of the ride. I'll say this for Evan: He knew how to change the subject.

The remainder of that evening was somewhat spoiled for me—I was afraid of the anger Evan had expressed and angry at what I had experienced as his disrespect for a man I had recently come to realize I loved. I spent that evening and all of the next day nervous, irritable, and discontented, unable to enjoy the normal weekend activities we had planned with Roger's extended family. My magnifying mind was working double shifts, trying to figure out exactly what was "wrong with this kid," and how I could set things right.

I thought about our conversation non-stop and picked apart his words, his gestures, and his tone of voice. I began to feel proud of myself. I had this kid and his problems all figured out, all right. Then why did I still feel like hell?

This feeling extended into the next day, a day during which I prayed, called my sponsor who was temporarily unavailable due to a grandchild's serious illness, attended my daily home group meeting, and did a fair day's work. Still, I was truly "restless, irritable, and discontented." Nothing I did took my mind off the events of the previous evening. It wasn't until a full twenty-four hours and at least one more meeting later, at four in the afternoon, while taking a smoke outside my office and thinking about Evan and *his* problems, that it hit me. "Oh," I thought. "I need to take my inventory and stop taking Evan's." This simple Tenth Step practice, had I done it as soon as I found myself disturbed by someone else's behavior, as the program suggests, could have saved me a very uncomfortable day and a half, during which I might have discovered the reasons for my discomfort in my own behavior by looking at my part in the disturbance.

What was my part in Evan's outburst? Well, to start with, I was in love with his father. Thinking of my own teenage years, I remembered how uncomfortable it made me to see any displays of affection between "old" people, especially between my parents—and they were *married* to each other! How awful it would have been to see either one of them with a different partner. I could have been a lot more considerate in Evan's presence in the past few weeks. I could have been a lot more discreet, especially since I realized, a bit belatedly, the day of Evan's explosion was the fifth anniversary of his biological mother's death.

My inventory helped me question what it must have felt like for a fourteen-year-old boy, who essentially was an only child, to see his father being openly affectionate with a woman who was not his mother on the anniversary of that mother's death. Not too good, I imagined. When I saw my part in what had happened in the car that evening, I was able to discuss this subject with Roger and modified my behavior accordingly. I was able to begin to show more sensitivity toward his son, explaining to Evan that I was not in his life in order to replace his mother, but to be his father's girlfriend and, in time, perhaps his wife, and that I would try to be a good friend to Evan, whatever happened between his father and me. Things got better between us. A few months later, the results of my changed approach became very clear.

Evan and I had discovered a shared love of cooking. One day in the kitchen, he left a pot with its handle hanging over the front of the stove. By this time, he had met and become friendly with the young men who would soon be his stepbrothers. We had shared backyard get-togethers and birthday parties as a family. On the day I noticed the pot handle sticking out dangerously over the edge of the stove, I couldn't help myself—I told Evan the same thing I'd told my other sons when they left a pot in that position: "This is dangerous, honey. Always make sure you leave a hot pot on the stove with its handle toward the back, so it doesn't get knocked over and hurt someone." Evan gave me one of those "Jeez, do you think I have brain damage?" looks fourteen-year-olds are so good at giving, but only for the briefest of seconds. "I'm sorry," I said as I winced. "I guess I just can't help being a mom." Evan's look of disdain evaporated, and he said (melting my heart), "Well, you're doing a pretty good job of that—with *two* families!" That was a "wow" moment for me. By taking my own inventory instead of his, and focusing on the only person I could change, myself, I opened the way for Evan and me to find our own stepmother-stepson relationship. By applying the principles of *The Soul Workout* to the best of my ability in our shared home, I had helped him move from a place of anger to a place of love. He and I share a special friendship and are moving toward a very special relationship as stepmother and stepson today.

Even though I try to remember to work the program of recovery in every aspect of my life, "sometimes the saddle slips," as my cowboy friend Mel says. Although I do my best to live in the program, sometimes I forget what I need to do. I forget to live in Steps Ten, Eleven, and Twelve, and sometimes it takes me time to remember that there is a solution, and it is in the Twelve Steps.

When I did my inventory in this case, I found that once I stopped trying to figure out what was "wrong" with Evan and looked at my own part in our evening's adventure, the feeling of "restlessness, irritability, and discontent" started to ooze away and was replaced with a feeling of serenity and goodwill.

In addition to seeing my part in what had happened in this particular instance, I learned an important life lesson that serves me inside and outside the rooms of recovery today: "Put yourself in someone else's shoes." In all relationships, even in fleeting and momentary transactions, I need to put myself quickly in the other party's place. Anyone I meet on any given day might be having the worst day of his or her life. I need to remember to treat everyone according to "principles, not personalities," as my program teaches. And I need to remember to do *The Soul Workout* to the best of my ability every day.

It always takes two to tango.
When you find yourself resenting someone
or something, take the time to step back and
identify your part in the situation.

When someone seems to upset you
for no good reason, consider that maybe
there's something about yourself that upsets
you for the same reason. **Accepting others with
their small "flaws" sometimes allows us to
accept our own annoying ways.** Accepting
ourselves as we are doesn't mean allowing
ourselves to behave unacceptably.

Gossip feeds resentments, so don't do it.
Ask your Higher Power for insight into
your own heart instead.

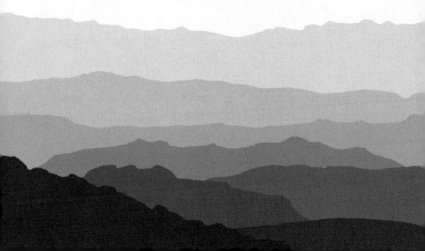

RIGOROUS HONESTY VS. SELF-INDULGENCE

Checking My Motives

About a year and a half into my recovery, and about three years into my widowhood, before I had met, heard of, or even knew Roger existed, I heard a fellowship member speak from the podium at a Saturday night twelve-step meeting. He was good-looking, smart, funny, and in recovery. And good-looking. Did I mention he was good-looking? I liked what I saw and what I heard. Until that time, I had followed the advice of my sponsor and other program friends—for the first year, I concentrated on my recovery and avoided getting into a relationship. To be honest, back then my disease had destroyed my looks to the point that it was not difficult to avoid romantic entanglements. But I felt ready. Actually, I felt over-ready.

The good-looking speaker's name was Conrad. When I shook his hand and thanked him after the meeting, he asked my name, which was not usual behavior from a visiting speaker. My sponsor, Joyce, who was standing next to me waiting to shake his hand, made eyes at me as if to say, "He likes you."

As we left the meeting hall, I told Joyce I liked him, too, and asked her advice. She suggested asking program friends about him and maybe finding out where he regularly attended meetings. That way we could go there too, and see if we could "run into" him again. Naturally, I would let my Higher Power handle it from there. After all, I'm in the footwork business, and my Higher Power is in the results business—that's what lots of people in recovery told me. So that's what I did.

Some of the friends we consulted were reluctant to speak negatively about Conrad, but a few hinted that he was a player. I didn't listen. It wasn't that I thought, "I can change him." It was that I thought, "They could be wrong," because I really wanted them to be. In retrospect, I realized I was acting impulsively instead of remaining open-minded and teachable.

My sponsor and I started attending the meetings Conrad went to, and to my surprise, he always made a beeline to sit next to me or across the table from me. Flirting ensued. The first time he passed me a note, I passed one right back as soon as Joyce's back was turned, knowing she would not have condoned this activity. I told myself I couldn't help it. I know that was not good meeting etiquette, but I was smitten—not to say getting desperate—and chose to not resist. After a few weeks of this sixth-grade behavior, I had had enough. It was time, I thought, to act like a grown-up woman instead of a middle school girl. I finally turned to Conrad, as the meeting was breaking up, and said:

> "So, um, Conrad…would you um…have… any…er…interest in seeing me…in a sort of non- meeting-type-of-situation? At all?"

He threw back his head and laughed, probably at the faltering way I asked, but who cares why? I had the chance to see that smile and those teeth. He said yes, and invited me to breakfast after the meeting. Over the next month there were phone calls, more post-meeting breakfasts, and a lunch or two. Not once did he make a move on me physically, and I wondered about that, but I ignored it. I was just happy to be the one looking at his beautiful golden eyes and to be the cause of the smile that crinkled his eyes at the corners.

True, he seemed to have many rules governing things like acceptable topics of conversation, but I didn't care; I was getting lost. He talked. I listened. He had a lot to say, which was fine, except when I wanted to say something. It finally dawned on me that I could not get a sentence into one of our "conversations" using the Jaws of Life. But I didn't mind too much. I was looking into his golden eyes and forgetting who I was. I tallied up the positives: He had a job. He had a car. He had a residence. And the last two of those items were separate things, which made him quite a catch in fellowship terms!

Conrad and I finally did go out together, and again it was because I spoke up first. In this case what I said was, "I want to go on a date with you." Yes, I had to be that specific.

Him: "What did you have in mind?"

Me: "Oh, I don't know, let me see...something wild and exotic. Like dinner and a movie."

Him: "Wild and exotic? That's American Standard!"

Me: "Well, you suggest something."

So we decided on a concert, with dinner first. I got a pedicure. I drove there in my own car, since it was our first "nighttime" date. I was excited. And it was awful.

He complained about the service at dinner, talked nonstop about himself, and sighed audibly throughout the show, at the end of which he stood up, looked at his watch, and said, "Well, that's two hours of my life I'll never get back." When we walked out to the parking lot, me trailing behind him, instead of walking me to my car, he put on his jacket, zipped it up, and practically left skid marks getting away from me. It was like one of those horror movies where one character sees the big scary monster behind the other character and runs away screaming. To say I was humiliated, frustrated, disappointed, and furious would really be an understatement.

Needless to say, Conrad didn't call to see if I got home okay. He didn't call the next day. Or the next. He seemed to have stopped attending his usual meetings, the ones where he had been running into me. It was evident that he had absolutely no further interest in me and that he hadn't even when we went on our "date" that night—not even in seeing that I got home safely. I was gravely disappointed, embarrassed, and hurt.

I worked out all those feelings in my fellowship, using the tools of the program, doing inventories, throwing myself into service, sharing at closed women's meetings, and talking and listening to my sponsor and other women friends. Time passed. I deleted Conrad's number from my phone, stopped going to the meetings he attended, and started going to different meetings. Of course, that might have been my Higher Power's plan for me all along. After a few months, when I was no longer feeling so ashamed and embarrassed, I met, got to know, and then quite unexpectedly entered a serious relationship with a different man. I didn't see Conrad again. Until about six weeks after I had become deeply involved with Roger.

It was at 7:00 a.m. one day when I had come directly from Roger's house. I was feeling suffused with love, when there, in the middle of the room at an early morning meeting, looking right at me, was the man I had come to think of as the Dreaded Conrad. He was smiling at me with those straight, white, even teeth and those golden eyes that crinkle at the corners when he smiles. After the reading, the sharing, and the closing prayer, he sought me out. I was sure my heart's thumping was audible. He spoke. "How's the writing going?" he asked, as if I had just been talking to him about it the day before. "Did you ever finish that book you were working on?" Blah, blah, blah.

I was distracted, dismayed, and excited. "Okay, Helen," I said to myself. "Just when you think you've divested yourself of any interest in seeing other men, and when you've told Roger you love him, and he's desperately in love with you, you see this guy who wiped the floor with you, and you're intrigued. Admit it; you know you are! What's the matter with you? Better yet, what is your Higher Power trying to teach you?"

I asked myself that question because that's what my sponsor always asks herself when life gets all "life-y" on her. If I follow her lead and start with the assumption that no matter what happens to me, my Higher Power's hand is in it, and He's trying to teach me something that will make me stretch and grow, I can handle most of my life's situations. An equally important thing for me to remember is that my Higher Power doesn't tempt. I don't know if there is a Lower Power, but if there is, I think tempting would be one of his jobs. I have to remember when I'm confronted with a tempting situation that my Higher Power's will for me will always lead me to growth and happiness, not into misery, confusion, or despair. As I pondered what could be happening here, and what my Higher Power wanted from me in this situation, Conrad and I walked out of the meeting side-by-side.

"I'll walk you to your car," he said, after we had stood and chatted for a moment or two with some other group members. I thought, "Well, that's more than you did the last time I saw you," and we walked together to my car. I was aware all the while of the absurdity of my wanting to spend more time in the company of this man I told myself I had written off as a bad actor, and of my hypocrisy in wanting him to find me as attractive as I'd found him months ago, and—let's face it—still did. I opened the door of my car and put my knapsack into the passenger seat, turned to face Conrad, smiled, put out my hand to shake his, took a deep breath to still my heart, and said, "I'm so glad to see you, especially since the last time I saw you, you were running away from me."

Him (*feigning shock*): "Running away?"

Me (*feigning toughness*): "Yeah. After the concert."

Him: "*You* said the only reason you were there that night is that your sponsor said…"

Me: "Go on, blame the victim."

While Conrad looked down at me disbelievingly, I told him that while it was true that I wouldn't have been out on a date with him if my sponsor hadn't encouraged me, I had been there because I *wanted* to be. I told him that I remembered what I had said, but that I couldn't argue with what he had heard. The conversation fizzled out after that, so I said good-bye. As I drove away, my heart was pounding. I called my sponsor to tell her about what had happened and to get her advice on how to handle the turmoil I was feeling.

She listened carefully, then said, "I think it was good that you laid it on the line with Conrad; and I notice that instead of saying, 'Yeah, I acted like a jerk; I'm sorry,' he just kind of turned it around on you. He justified himself by pointing out where he thought you were wrong. Ask yourself, would Roger do that? I don't think so. Is that what the Tenth Step tells us to do? I don't think so."

She was right.

The rest of that day when Conrad first reappeared was rough. Even though I was certain of my feelings for and responsibility to Roger, and knew Conrad had treated me badly (and would be certain to do so again, given half a chance, judging by his inability to speak a simple, unadorned "I'm sorry"), I found myself thinking about Conrad all day. Was it possible that he had gotten even *better* looking in the intervening months? Was it a coincidence that he turned up in a meeting I attended in an obscure part of town? Would it be possible to start over again with him? Thoughts like these cycled through my head and repeated themselves all day. Then, to make matters worse, as I was leaving a meeting that evening where I had just shared about this very subject, who was among the people waiting to get into the room for the next meeting? CONRAD. I was unnerved to see him, and then he saw me. Then I was *really* unnerved.

Him: "Wow. Twice in one day…"

Me: (*trying to sound tough*) "That's 'cause you're stalking me."

I said this very slowly, trying to appear sassy and nonchalant, and scrunched myself up to squeeze past him in the too-narrow passageway, trying hard not to touch him, which might have let him feel how hard I was shaking. "Try to saunter," I told myself, "and don't look back." I made it to my car and sat for a few minutes, just breathing. "You did good," I assured myself. But all night this scene played in the back of my mind. It intruded on my time with Roger that evening, and I debated inwardly whether to tell Roger about it or not.

What does "rigorous honesty" demand? I asked myself. Does it mean I should ease my mind by discussing every thought about everything with my partner, even if to do so might interfere with his peace of mind? How would I feel if the situation were reversed? Would I want to know that Roger had run into an old girlfriend who had stirred up feelings that day? Just what does the program mean when it demands "rigorous honesty"? Does it mean I can never have private thoughts and feelings? What would Joyce say about this?

That last question was the key, of course. With time in recovery and a good working relationship with a sponsor, a recovering person often knows what that sponsor would say on certain topics without even asking. Don't get me wrong; it's still critically important to ask. The action of doing so is important for my growth. I cannot assume I know what's best for me—considering that my own thoughts and actions got me to the lowest point of my life before I entered recovery. I can see Joyce's face and hear her voice even when she's not with me, but that is not license to "sponsor myself."

True honesty enables me to admit that I know right from wrong today, just like any other moral adult human being. I don't always need an outside advisor for that because I have a conscience today, and it's a healthy one, thanks to my program and my fellowship of recovery. I can wait, sometimes, until the time is right, to share with my sponsor or a trusted program friend, or I can write about whatever is troubling me until I can discuss it with Joyce or another woman in the program. And I was pretty certain what Joyce would have told me to do that night.

She would have asked me to examine my motives in wanting to tell Roger about this nonevent. Would I really be practicing "rigorous honesty," or would I be selfishly and self-centeredly boosting my own ego by rubbing Roger's nose in the fact that I had lingering feelings about another man—even one whom I'd written off as unsuitable long, long ago—and enjoyed knowing this other man still wanted to at least flirt with me? What character defect was at work here? Most likely vanity, which is one of my top ten and arises from insecurity and, in my case, comes from fear—fear of being less-than, fear of not getting enough attention, affection, or adulation. In other words, this is all about ego.

I ran through the possible results that would ensue if I spoke my mind. Every one of them ended with Roger being unnecessarily troubled by my mere thoughts about a man whom I knew I would not be happy with and had no intention of pursuing, though I'm sure he possessed many terrific qualities, including those eyes and that smile.

After an evening in which I maintained my silence on the subject, I did call Joyce. I didn't mention my inner thoughts to Roger at that time. After all, even addicts who are trying to live honestly may have private thoughts and feelings, especially ones that might cause unnecessary anxiety to those who love them. The important thing for me to keep in mind is always my motive. I have to remember that there is rigorous honesty, and then there is brutal honesty. While my program teaches that it's important to "tell on ourselves" at the group level or with a sponsor, the most important person I need to be honest with is myself. This is especially important in discerning my motives in every situation and examining my actions or projected actions for traces of the character defects of fear, resentfulness, selfishness, and dishonesty. When I do this, I learn the truth about myself, and I build my soul.

Once I spoke with Joyce, wrote down my feelings about this non-incident, and put my trust in the process, I was able to lighten up, stop taking myself so seriously, and talk about it with Roger. I was able to be completely honest in a way that didn't disturb or unnerve him and that helped me to feel closer to him, which is one of the goals of *The Soul Workout* for me—to be able to treat others in my life with respect, dignity, and love, as I would want to be treated. I need to be honest with others about my thoughts, feelings, and actions, but first, I must be honest with myself. Doing this consistently, seeking the vision of God's will for me in all I say and do each day, being as honest and transparent as I possibly can, is one of the ways I grow my soul.

For much of my life before I entered recovery, I couldn't handle the truth about myself, or, as one of my home group brothers says, I couldn't handle "my own authenticity." My program of recovery demands rigorous honesty, and as an addict, I'm by nature the sort of person who lies when the truth would serve her better. Honesty is something I had to cultivate and practice in recovery, both in and out of twelve-step meeting rooms.

Practicing the principles of my twelve-step program has given me the tools to look at my motives to the best of my ability in every situation and to uncover, discover, and discard some hard truths about myself. But unless I use these tools, I cannot become the person I know my Higher Power wants me to be.

Don't tell lies, except when people
ask you if their pants make them look fat.
What are they going to do, go home and change?
Tell them they look fine. To God, they do.

Say you're talking to your lover, and you
are asked a question, and the truthful answer
might hurt. Say it anyway, but say it with love.
**The truth may hurt, but it will not harm the
way a lie will.** No good can come from a lie.
No real harm can come from the truth.

**Don't call an old person "young lady" or
"young man."** They know it's not true,
and at their age they've earned the respect of not
being mocked. They already know they're old;
just "sir" or "ma'am" will suffice.

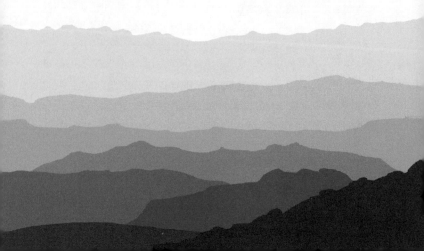

SPIRITUALITY

Filling My God Hole

My second husband, John, died at the age of fifty-one from the chronic, progressive, and fatal brain disease of addiction. He and I had had a truly symbiotic addict/codependent/enabler relationship. We used day and night, together and separately, for the entirety of the brief time we had with each other. My marriage to John couldn't have been more different from my relationship with my first husband, Sal. Sometimes I think Sal's disapproval was the only thing that kept me alive long enough to get into recovery the first time, at the age of forty. Using while being married to Sal had been like trying to drive a car with the emergency brake on—I still got to where I wanted to go, but only with great difficulty and a lot of dedicated effort.

In my first marriage, my addiction, along with social-drinking Sal's corresponding codependence, had been a major and entirely misunderstood factor in the turbulence and unhappiness he and I lived with for far too many years. Sal was not an addict; however, my addiction and his codependence destroyed any chance we ever had for a meaningful or truly loving relationship. Yet we lasted almost thirty years together, grinding our teeth and white-knuckling it most of the way. It was not a relationship in which spirituality played any part.

Even when I entered recovery toward the end of that first marriage, my grasp of and commitment to twelve-step recovery was weak. At that time, all I had was physical abstinence. There was no spiritual growth. I had made the mistake many do and thought that if I just didn't use and attended meetings, I could undo the damage I'd done over so many years. I also believed that since Sal had desperately wanted me to quit using for so long, the simple fact of my quitting would have been sufficient to keep him happy. I wasn't working a program of recovery. I was attending meetings and not using, and that was it. Needless to say, it was a shock to me to find myself divorced six years into what I then called recovery, rejected in favor of an older woman (ouch!). All-too-quickly I embarked on a "get-better" relationship with the man who would become my second husband—John—within a year of my divorce. Looking back, I can see that I was using sex and love addictively, getting a fix from a man who genuinely did love me, but who was also hell-bent on his own destruction from this disease. Once again, spirituality was absent entirely from my life and from John's.

The night John and I became a couple, I was not using and hadn't been for years. I cannot say I was in recovery, but I was alcohol-free, and that was it. I had smoked pot occasionally and told myself that since it wasn't alcohol, my favored substance of abuse, I was okay. I had stopped attending meetings or doing any type of service work in my fellowship. I never really worked the steps. Reading them off the wall at meetings is no substitute for working them with a sponsor. In addition to doing it my way, I never gave the slightest thought to seeking the "spiritual awakening" the program calls for. As a result, I had no adequate defense against picking up my drug of choice.

Within a month after John and I got together, I was in Louie's Basque restaurant in Reno on a business trip, ordering (of all things) a Campari and soda. "What's the harm in a little Italian liqueur?" was my reasoning, as far as there was any reasoning at all going on. The harm, I saw only long afterward, was that one rather wimpy little drink triggered the phenomenon of craving, and because the disease of addiction is fatal and progressive, I soon surpassed the degree of using that had brought me into recovery six years earlier. When John and I married—eight months after I took that first drink and almost a year after that joint—I was in full-blown addiction once again. Our marriage, which was fun, hopeful, and loving at first, soon disintegrated into a hell of injuries, illness, filth, degradation, and despair.

We had been married about three years when John was hospitalized for the first time with pancreatitis. This was followed by two months of intensive care, expensive medical treatment, and inpatient physical rehabilitation in a series of nursing homes. He returned home in a wheelchair. He had a feeding tube in his stomach, which I was expected to learn how to clean and use to feed him. During one lucid interval while he was recovering physically from his hospital stay, I asked John if he had any fear of death, knowing that he was an avowed atheist. He turned the question around on me:

"Were *you* afraid before you were born?"

"No…"

"Well, then why should you be afraid of what happens after you die?"

I thought then that he had a good point, and in some ways, I still do. One of the main elements of my childhood belief in God was fear of death and what came (or didn't come) afterward. My mother had instilled in me a terror of being sent to "the bad fire." She even went so far as to show me, down in the basement of the pre-World War II apartment building where we lived in New York, the monstrous furnace-boiler complex, making sure I got a good look at the open door of the firebox, to ensure I understood what spending an eternity wrapped in flames would look like.

John had no such fear. He was a complete and strong, or positive, atheist. He actively rejected belief in a deity, unlike some, called in philosophy weak or negative atheists, who simply do not believe there is a God. The distinction is subtle and can be difficult to discern for some; but ultimately, John was an atheist, meaning he had no belief in a deity. He lived, feeling neither the need for God nor the fear of God. John was one of the most highly intelligent, devastatingly sexy, rakishly handsome, hilariously funny, and completely alcoholic men I've ever met. He also was one of the most spiritually dead people I've ever known.

I believed—and naturally, my belief was colored by love—that John was as moral a person as an addicted person can be. He knew right from wrong and often tried his best to do right. He respected the beliefs of others, and he was able to love, albeit in a limited way. I've learned in twelve-step recovery that it is not necessary to believe in a deity in order to be spiritual. Atheism, in my opinion, can be a very spiritual state of being. It depends on the atheist. However, John neither believed in a deity, nor was he spiritually fit. He just was completely shut down as far as his relationship with a Higher Power was concerned. God did not ping on John's radar.

All my life I've wanted to be tough and cool, like John. I really *wanted* to be an atheist, but I had a problem. I had a "God hole," although I didn't know that's what it was called. I just knew there was something inside me that needed and wanted a relationship with God, and I hated that part of myself—so weak, so needy, and so vulnerable. The part of me that has always wanted and needed a relationship with God is the part of me that I have always tried to deny even exists. It needs so much, and I hated admitting

I needed anything. I'm also terrified that I won't get whatever I bring myself to admit I need. I wanted to be like John, who was seemingly so tough, cool, self-sufficient, and completely self-contained. Sadly, he also was completely addicted and truly powerless and ignorant of his powerlessness. I could never admit that I really wanted and needed a relationship with a Higher Power. I was actually ashamed of this need, so I wanted to deny that a Higher Power could even exist. I was a mess.

I did exactly what seemed right to me, in my distorted manner of thinking, in falling in love with and marrying a person in active addiction. That decision brought me to this point—straddling my husband's still-cooling corpse in a pool of blood, screaming his name as loud as I could, and slapping his face with all my strength. I was drunk by the time the coroner arrived an hour later, and I stayed that way for two years.

When I reentered recovery, two years after John died at home in my arms on a Thursday morning, I knew enough from my previous attempt at recovery to know that I needed to get a sponsor right away, and I did. She didn't allow me to languish in idleness. She had almost twenty years in the program at that time and knew that I would find relief in the steps. So she started me working on them right away.

Only God can fill a God hole. I've tried filling my God hole with other things, and for a while it seemed to work. When I start to feel the pounding, aching emptiness inside that yells, "Fill me. Now!" I start to scramble, seeking frantically that one thing that will do the trick. "Him.""That.""More." They all work, for a little while. Until they don't.

Until I figured out that what I had was a God hole, and that I'd been trying to fill that hole with everything from men to shoes to shiny objects, I had no hope of ever filling that hole in a way that would stop the pounding and stop the ache. Today I know that what I need is God. The best way to remain connected to my God is through prayer, meditation, and service to His other children.

Visit the sick. Trust me, everyone gets
depressed by hospitals; you are not unique.
The sick person is much more depressed by
being in the hospital than you are by visiting it.

When you give change to homeless people,
look them in the eye. If they say, "Thank you,"
make sure you say, "You're welcome."
They are giving you more than you are giving
them—**an opportunity to build your soul.**

Learn and practice prayer and meditation.
Ask your Higher Power daily to guide
you according to His or Her will.
Believe that "if God brings you to it,
He will bring you through it."

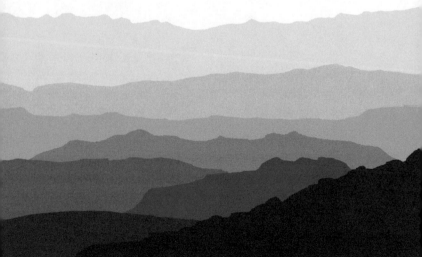

GRIEF AND LOSS

Learning to Heal through Tears and Love

My sponsor, Joyce, introduced me to a women's meeting group the first week she and I started working together as sponsor and sponsee. One of the other women members of the group was a delightful fellow redhead named Elaine. She had been Joyce's sponsee for several years by the time we met, and her wild, yet entirely feminine, laughter and her open, adorable smile carried me through many an early pitfall in my first days in recovery. While there were times, when I was being a "typical newcomer," she might have been laughing *at* me, it always seemed like she was laughing *with* me. She was loving, caring, and encouraging—a true "sponsister," as we called each other. From her and from Joyce I learned how to be a woman among women in recovery, how to laugh and cry together, how to fulfill responsibilities cheerfully, how to show up for life and for other people, and how to have fun, too.

A few months into our friendship, Elaine began to mention abdominal pains that wouldn't go away. Her doctor seemed to think the problem was digestive, and treated her accordingly. Elaine had abused alcohol during her active addiction, and when she was unable to obtain drinking alcohol, she would resort to isopropyl, vanilla extract, or mouthwash. The idea that she would have residual stomach problems years after entering recovery was not so far-fetched. Brief periods of relief would be followed by longer and longer periods of pain, until finally the awful diagnosis was made: uterine cancer. The months and months of misdiagnoses had made it certain that the disease had metastasized, and Elaine's prognosis was dire.

Back before Elaine knew she was so sick, when my first anniversary in recovery had arrived, our sponsor, Joyce, was in a wheelchair with a broken leg. The group in which I hoped to mark my recovery birthday was one that shared a cake with each celebrant. The obvious choice of who would present my first birthday cake to me would have been my sponsor; however, since Joyce was out of commission, Elaine took on that task enthusiastically and energetically. Unbelievably, six months later she would be dead.

Joyce and I told each other that Elaine had died *with* the disease of addiction; she did not die *from* it, and that was some comfort. As it is for most people who lose a friend or family member in what should have been his or her prime of life, it was hard for me to believe Elaine was no longer with us. In fact, there were many times when I was certain I could feel her presence around me in the days and months after her death. This comforted me, but it made me angry, as well. You see, while I felt the presence of my recent friend, Elaine, I had never felt the presence of John, my husband, whom I had loved passionately. Why had I never felt his presence since his death? This thought depressed and tormented me.

He had died two years before Elaine, and I had never, ever felt even a glimmer of his presence since then, although I had dearly wanted to. I thought of him for hours every day, cried about him, wept when a song we had enjoyed together played on the radio, touched the things he had touched, and even wore the things he had worn, but nothing gave me a feeling of his presence. After entering recovery, I even prayed for him, but I felt nothing. It was as if, when he had died in my arms, he'd gone *out,* like a candle flame blown out by a gust of wind.

After losing my friend Elaine, I often remembered things she would say and the simple spiritual practices she would perform, such as when, before leaving her house in the morning or entering her car, she would hold the door open for a few seconds and center herself by saying, "God, You go first." I found myself imitating her in my early recovery, and after she died, these small rituals began to mean a great deal to me. I felt her presence most strongly when performing an action she taught me. Perhaps that's not surprising. Researchers have looked into the feeling of "presence," but of course cannot come to any conclusion. How can they? Science is designed to explain the natural world, not the world of the spirit.

Is the feeling of "presence" simply a manifestation of grief? Maybe. Is it an indication that the dead do live on spiritually and that we are able to sense them around us? Who knows? What I knew then was that I missed my husband, and I wished I had some ongoing sense of connectedness to him, like the one I experienced for my friend, Elaine.

This unsatisfied desire for connection was with me for most of the first year and a half of my recovery. I thought I grieved John at the time of his death, but since my active addiction actually accelerated after he died—after all, I was the bereaved widow—I realized I didn't really feel grief, much less any of my emotions. What I felt was a great sense of abandonment and a ton of self-pity. When the fog finally cleared at about a year and a half in recovery, I really began to feel grief for the first time. It was like a direct hit in the stomach with the blunt end of a pool stick.

One morning during this time of true grieving, while driving to my morning home group meeting, a song came on the radio that John and I had loved. We used to put it on and slow-dance to it in the living room. He would sing along with the music to me. It was a love song called *Stainsby Girl* and was written by a British artist for his wife. John would brush back my hair, kiss me, and whisper, "You're *my* wee Stainsby girl," as the music played and we held each other. As the song played again on the radio in my car, I remembered those moments and began to weep, and continued to weep quietly as I parked the car and entered the meeting place.

Tears in a twelve-step meeting are not unusual, especially when we are new. We have a lot to cry about—tears of remorse, of sadness, of regret. Then, when we have been in recovery for a while, we may cry tears of joy or gratitude. So I wasn't ashamed or embarrassed as I took my seat, and although my friends looked at me with concern as the meeting got under way, I was able to shake my head and smile weakly to indicate that these tears were okay, and so was I.

One of the reasons I selected my home group is because it focuses on "the solution." Our meeting format consists of an opening prayer, greetings, and a welcome to newcomers and out-of-town visitors, followed by a reading from our recovery book, then by sharing, with each member who shares "tagging," or calling on, another member, who may choose to share or pass. As I listened to the reading that morning, I looked around the room at the faces of the people who had once been no more than friendly strangers to me, but who had become my spiritual family. We were all diverse recovering members getting better collectively, held together by the mysterious forces of gratitude, fellowship, and love, but it can't be denied that there were distinct "personalities" in the room that tended to draw members into smaller, discrete "grouplets."

At one table, dubbed the "AARP Table," some old-timers who had been members of the fellowship for anywhere from fifteen to thirty years had coalesced into a loosely knit formation of "elders," and who could be counted on for their wisdom. Another table, called by some the "Arts & Crafts Table," featured a small cadre of gay men, one of whom usually works on an elegant piece of needlepoint while listening or sharing. This arrangement turned out to be enormously beneficial to gay newcomers who are able to gravitate to them and find comfort, safety, and examples of fellowship and recovery when they may need it most, before assimilating into the rest of the group, which they soon do.

At another table were young, and sometimes not-so-young, women residents of a nearby recovery home. It was something to watch the light come back on in their eyes, from when they entered recovery and would shuffle across the room to flop into their seats until a month or so later, when they began to hold their heads up and take pride in their appearance once again before reentering the world.

Then there was the table where I usually found my seat. We were the "Odds and Ends Table," composed of a loose core of regulars who had no discernible affiliation other than friendship and love. Around the walls of the room sat old-timers, newcomers, and out-of-town visitors, along with some homeless people and some people who were well-to-do. The back of the room was usually where the men from various halfway houses sat, interspersed with a gaggle of regulars and visitors from other groups. Everyone was welcome, and there were no hard-and-fast rules about who sat where. All of us were attached to one another by the bonds of fellowship and a shared conviction that we were here to save our lives.

As I sat at the Odds and Ends Table and listened to the reading and then the sharing, my heart swelled with love for my home group members. It was a love that was mixed with a piercing sadness as I reflected that John never found recovery. As I mused tearfully on this, the conviction began to grow in me that perhaps the reason I felt no connection with John was that there was nothing to feel a connection to—that he truly no longer existed. I saw clearly, for the first time, that his soul, so weak to begin with, never sheltered or nourished during all the fifty-one years of his difficult and sometimes painfully miserable life, once freed from his body, had nowhere to live. John was gone.

It was then and there that the idea of *The Soul Workout* really began to take shape. The whitewashed church hall, lit by fluorescent lights that sometimes flickered or buzzed, furnished with tables and chairs that were chipped or wobbly, with a tired linoleum floor that dipped treacherously in some places and buckled in others, was the room in which I had entered recovery. My very first meetings had taken place here, and it was here I'd taken my first faltering steps into the fellowship that had not only saved my life, but that had given me a life *worth* saving, as my friend Ty often said. Here I began, by imitation, to build my own soul, following the examples around me. My spiritual fitness had grown to the extent that I had worked the program, in this room, in rooms like it, and in my everyday life. I had become aware of the difference between spiritual fitness and spiritual unfitness, and it was like the difference between life and death. I knew I felt different here than I had at any other time in my life. I also knew that as much as I'd loved him, I'd never felt this way when John and I were dancing our dance of death together. Neither one of us had the least bit of interest in our souls and their fitness, and, in fact, would have laughed at anyone who attempted to interest us in our spiritual health or lack thereof. As long as we had our drug of choice, we were as spiritually alive as we thought we wanted to be. And mostly, we wanted to be oblivious.

As I sat in that meeting on that particular day, my thoughts were less on the speakers and more on John and his death. I recalled that awful morning when I came to from my stupor of the previous evening and it *finally* dawned on me that my husband was dying in front of me, only a few feet away. He had hemorrhaged the night before, after drinking some whiskey I'd brought home for my own consumption and begrudgingly shared with him. The blood was still everywhere, since I had been too loaded even to make an effort to clean it up the previous night. There was so much blood, as Lady Macbeth once observed of another Scotsman.

As I'd foggily begun to realize what was happening, I picked up the living room phone to call my job to tell them I was taking John back to the hospital and that I wouldn't be in to work. Before I finished the call, he struggled manfully, sat upright, and faced me, one arm pointing toward me, index finger extended. It was as if he saw something I couldn't see—something near me, but invisible. Then his arm dropped slowly to his side and he began to slide toward me, off the sofa where he'd slept the night before, the last night of his life on earth.

I dropped the phone receiver and leaped across the room to him, a distance of three or four feet, but I cleared it easily. By this time he had slid completely off the sofa, his knees folding under him, causing him to assume a kneeling posture, and about to topple forward as the strength left his body. I jumped the distance between us, managed to straddle him, and got my arms under his, holding him up, listening to his last breaths and barely able to comprehend what was happening. Last night's hemorrhage was evident everywhere, on him, on me, on the furniture, and on the floor. I held John as life left him. It is quite a thing to hold the difference between life and death in your arms. There was no rattle, simply a cessation of breathing, and then he went slack. I drew one arm from around him and slapped his face, hard, then harder. I shouted his name again and again. Then, after interminable moments, stunned, panicked, unable to hold even his pitifully emaciated frame upright any longer, I let my husband's body slide onto the floor, where his head came to rest, and the blackish blood that had pooled inside him ran out, through his nostrils, to mingle with what he had bled the night before.

A long night began for me then, a night of loneliness, misery, and despair. It would be a full two years before dawn broke, in the form of recovery. In recovery, I regained my dignity, my womanhood, and my life. I would never forget John, but I knew I did not want a death like his. In recovery, I get to choose the way I live and, to a certain extent, the way I will die. I don't know when or how death will take me, but I do know this: As long as I use the simple tools of my program and remain spiritually fit, I will die, like Elaine, with the disease of addiction, not from it.

On September 11, 2001, I awoke to images of the Twin Towers, which my father, a bricklayer, had helped erect in the late sixties and early seventies. That morning the towers were burning and would soon fall. Like the rest of the world, I was fixed on my TV screen, watching the horror unfold. Amid the smoke billows, flecks of white began to swirl through the air. The towers had been full of offices, and offices are full of paper, paper that made ready fuel to feed the fires that were bringing the structures down, and some of which was escaping like horrid confetti over lower Manhattan. There was something else, too, something more horrid still. Human forms began to be discernible through the smoke; tiny, doll-like figures, some singly, some in pairs, began to appear at what was left of the windows—stranded too high for rescuers to reach, they had a split-second to decide how they wanted to die, consumed in a fireball or broken on the sidewalk a thousand feet below. Those who jumped chose the sidewalk.

Like those who jumped from the towers and those who didn't, and like everyone else on earth, I will die someday. Recovery doesn't change that. Death is not my enemy; losing my recovery is.

Today, I identify with those tiny figures in the smoke on that terrible September morning. Faced with impending death, they exercised the only choice left to them. They chose the way they preferred to die. By doing what I need to do to stay in recovery, I get to choose the way I will die, as well as the way I will live. I choose to live free, honest, and spiritually fit. I choose a life in recovery, and I choose not to die loaded—that's an ugly death, and it often takes innocent bystanders down with it. I have a choice today; I choose a life in recovery.

An old saying goes, "Never mention rope in the house of a man who's been hanged." **Be conscious of your listener's circumstances before you speak.** Has he or she been newly diagnosed with cancer, diabetes, or any other serious illness? Avoid mentioning your Aunt Jo who died of it. This sounds so commonsensical, but it's amazing how many of us, through lack of conscious consideration, make this mistake.

When you experience a significant loss— whether by death, divorce, illness, injury, or other circumstance—**give yourself the gift of feeling your grief,** whatever form it may take and however long it lasts.

Offer simple condolences like "I'm sorry for your loss." **You don't have to be a poet in order to help someone who is suffering feel comforted.**

YOU'RE READY WHEN YOU'RE READY

Stumbling toward Recovery

I was sixteen years old in the summer of 1969, going to summer school to make up for the math class I failed during the year and working as a cashier in a supermarket in Jamaica, Queens. I was dating the boy who would become my first husband, and during that time I was an addict who hadn't had my first drug yet. Of course, as a child I sucked the foam off my daddy's beer, and when I was seven, some uncles visiting from Scotland thought it would be funny to get a little girl drunk on Guinness. That was my first drunk, and the first time I passed out on a hard, white bathroom floor, face down on the cool, octagonal tiles, only to come to at the sound of my mother's voice, yelling uselessly at her in-laws, who by then were too far gone to know what the hell she was mad about.

Because my father was an often-angry, unpredictable drunk, as I entered my teens I had an antipathy toward alcohol. I wouldn't become like him. That is not to say I wouldn't drink or use; I just wouldn't become like him. I would never throw any child of mine down a flight of stairs. I wouldn't come to and then vomit for an hour every morning before work. I wouldn't rage at my spouse, embarrass my family, ruin evenings out, make a martyr of anyone, argue with bewildered strangers, demand and then refuse food, or create soiled underwear that would then be hung on the laundry line by my spouse in a futile effort to embarrass me. I would never take off my belt to use it as a weapon, stab forks into kitchen tables, threaten to have my family deported, or make unfounded and malicious accusations against them. I would never drag my unwilling spouse away from his parents and family to settle in an unfamiliar country alone, and then abandon him while I drank myself angry, vicious, and sick. I would never wake up my thirteen-year-old from a sound sleep at two in the morning to drag her across town to baby-sit for a stranger's children in a strange house so the stranger and I could continue our barhopping. I would be present in my children's lives. I would take notice of them, and when I took them on Saturday morning outings, it wouldn't be to the Market Diner and Bar at the NY piers. I would never shame them, as my father did when I married that first boyfriend at the age of nineteen, walking me down the aisle like a drunken sailor, leaving me at the altar with a kiss, then turning left and bolting unsteadily out the sacristy door. The sounds of my father's vomiting made an interesting accompaniment to the organist's otherwise soulful version of *Ave Maria*.

The disease of addiction doesn't run in my family; it flies a B-52. Although I promised myself I'd never become a drunk like my father, I was determined to try drinking. What was it in those bottles that made them so irresistible to my grown-up relatives? As superior as

I felt to my father, as judgmental of his drinking, I was still dying to know. Part of being a grown-up in my family was either to drink, like my father and uncles, or to be a raging, untreated, codependent enabler, like my mother, my grandmother, and many of my aunts. The drunks looked like they were getting away with murder and having fun doing it, but the nondrinkers just looked angry, unhappy, and dull. I knew to which branch of the family I wanted to belong.

At the supermarket where I worked in the summer of '69, there were two other teenagers, a boy and a girl who were dating each other. Louis had a van, and Polly was in love with him. One Thursday in August 1969, she came up next to me as we waited to punch our timecards and said she and Louis were driving his van upstate the next day to a concert, and asked if my boyfriend and I would like to go, too. "Okay," I said. "I'll ask my parents." I think I must have been the only kid in history to ask her parents for permission to join a revolution.

When I got home that afternoon, my father was at the kitchen table reading the *Journal-American*, a newspaper big enough to obscure my view of his face. Just as well, since in those days my attire consisted of two handkerchiefs tied together to make a blouse, no bra, and a pair of jeans so well worn and covered with patches that there was very little of the original pair of jeans left. At that time I thought I was a funny-looking, too-smart, nearsighted girl with a space between her teeth and horn-rimmed glasses. I realize now that

I was, in those days, a green-eyed, gorgeous, sex-crazed, red-haired, half-naked, freckle-faced, sixteen-year-old, would-be-hippie chick, not exactly the kind of little girl that sets a father's heart at ease—more the kind that pushes a father into an early grave. So it was a good thing that just as I couldn't see him, he really couldn't see me, either.

"Daddy," I said, very quickly so I could get it all out and maybe get an answer from him before he had a chance to think, "Polly and Louis are going to a concert called Woodstock, and they're taking Louis's van, and they want to know if Sal and I can go with them…." A plume of cigarette smoke drifted up from behind my father's newspaper. He didn't even bend the page down to look at me.

"Aye," he answered, in his Scottish burr. "Can ye get there wi' two broken legs?"

There was some question in my mind in those days as to whether or not my father *would* actually commit grievous bodily harm upon me, and rightly so, as the stair-throwing incident was still in my future, so I wasn't certain he might not actually make good on that threat. And this is the story of how I never got to Woodstock.

As I write this, the fortieth anniversary of Woodstock has just passed. Members of my cohort, aging baby boomers, are nostalgic now and conversations turn to the events and activities of that long-ago time. When people in my life whose parents were either more permissive or less aware of what their kids were doing, or who as kids were either bolder, sneakier, or wilder than I was, talk about those days, my recovering self does feel a twinge of envy. There's a teenaged girl inside me still, and she sometimes wishes she had done more of what her peers did, and harbors a sliver of regret that she'll never be able to do those things now. My generation is so much associated with "sex, drugs, and rock 'n' roll" that I almost feel "less than" or "apart from" my peers who took more and different substances than I did—until I remember that addiction is not in the substance, it's in the person. It's in me. It doesn't really matter what I took or what I was too scared to take. In fact, my fears and timidity might have been what kept me alive long enough to enter recovery.

My fear of needles dates back to my emergency appendectomy at age nine, when the mean nurse with the Teutonic accent had trouble finding a vein for an IV and yelled at me as she stabbed repeatedly in the soft crook of my arm while my father held me rigid on his lap. Remembering this episode kept me far away from using injectable substances. Besides, as drugs infiltrated the American middle class in the sixties, I knew too many kids who were sitting next to me in the classroom one day, and were then dead of an overdose the next. Obviously, you either had to know what you were doing to shoot up or you had to be too wild to care, and I was just too scared of the needle to make even experimenting seem worthwhile.

Hallucinogenics held some interest, but even as a teenager I somehow knew I was never in the right frame of mind to drop acid. I was always too depressed, frightened, anxious, embarrassed, ashamed, despairing, neurotic, and generally messed-up for acid; and anyway, the only girl in my school who could have been a connection had the filthiest nails I'd ever seen in my life. Oh, I got weed from her, which she got from her equally filthy boyfriend, but the idea of ingesting anything even marginally more substantial than smoke that had passed through her possession somehow turned me off. I remember thinking, "I wouldn't swap lunches with her, never mind putting something she'd touched into my brain!" So acid was out.

With my red hair in two pigtails and my horn-rimmed glasses on my little, freckled nose, I looked like a farm-girl-ready-to-go-bad. I had enough of a "good girl" veneer that nobody would ever seriously offer me anything stronger than a hash-laced joint. My "drug of choice"—what a misnomer; like most addicts, I had very little choice in the matter—would remain alcohol. It was cheap, legal, and socially acceptable, within limits, of course.

I was always a fan of inhalants, though, and my friends would frequently remind me to rub the black (gasoline) or white (correction fluid) circles from the end of my nose. When I was diagnosed with asthma at the age of twenty-one, I was delighted to discover theophylline elixir, a kind of precursor of the energy-drink-and-vodka cocktail. Theophylline elixir was a clear, reddish blend of the bronchodilator theophylline in an alcohol-water suspension. It tasted vile, and went down with a shudder, but it got me where I wanted to go. Of course, I had to take a lot of it, which meant I had to fake a lot of asthma attacks. When I began to experience what I later learned were some of theophylline's side effects—lack of appetite and nausea—I was elated. While my friends were putting on weight, I was staying thin and energized. And loaded.

For years, I alternated between abusing theophylline and other prescribed asthma medications in pill form, which produced a delicious, exhilarating sense of agitation and a hyper-energetic effect, and prescription tranquilizers and sedatives, which I took whenever I could get them. I felt it was not often enough, but as a therapy patient for many years, I did manage to avail myself of whatever was on offer.

Marriage and young motherhood gave me the children I had always wanted, making it difficult for me to score anything but booze, which was always available, always legal, always there. Alcohol was the mainstay of my addiction for many, many years. My pregnancies were periods of abstinence, but my old-world parents believed that Guinness Stout was good for nursing mothers, and so once my sons were delivered and I was nursing, my parents brought me Guinness every time they visited, insisting that it would help my milk come down. Even with my parents providing me with alcohol and my Italian father-in-law's "hospitality" of pouring me a glass of wine, saying, "Here, you may as well be drunk as the way you are," I was still able to carry, deliver, nurse, and raise three healthy boys. My first husband's disapproval and the fact that I hadn't yet crossed "the invisible line" made it possible for me to maintain a level of abstinence that lasted well into the late days of my sons' childhoods.

Eventually, my addiction broke loose and roared ferociously through my thirties, and by the week of my fortieth birthday had reached previously unplumbed depths. After all, "the big four-oh" is a milestone for most people, even "normies," and my birthday is the day after St. Patrick's Day, a day when even normal people get loaded. Why wouldn't I? The week of that birthday, I don't think I drew a single unintoxicated breath. In those days, corporations were not as sensitive as they are now about drinking alcohol during office hours, and even responsible bosses would often bring in cases of beer for "after-work" celebrations that sometimes began at lunchtime. Everything was in place for a run of cataclysmic proportions, and I took full advantage of everything that I could.

St. Patrick's Day fell on a Tuesday that year. My birthday was on a Wednesday. That Saturday night, my husband Sal was to receive an award at a dinner dance for his years of service to his teacher's union. No surprise that I was so drunk I embarrassed him and everyone around me, ending the evening by confronting the wife of one of his coworkers. I pointed my finger at her and said, "Fuck you. You're just a privileged white woman in a fur hat!" I blacked out soon after, but I remember the feel of my exasperated and humiliated husband's hand as it clamped down on the back of my neck. I have a hazy memory of pouting in the passenger seat of our car with my arms crossed, freezing in the New York City March night, as he drove us home in silent rage.

I came to the next day in an empty house—no husband in the bed next to me, no children watching television downstairs. Not even a note. What little recall I had of the events from the previous week, and especially the previous night, was blurred; but the moments that remained clear to me were disgusting and degrading. That's all my story ever was. There were no dramatic arrests, no heart-wrenching child-protective services involvement, no high-speed car chases, no DUIs, no humiliating firings. It was just pure and utter degradation.

I came to on that Sunday morning swimming in a pool of sweat, alone, unable to stop the painful twitching in my limbs, and when I managed to get upright enough to lurch to the bathroom, I didn't know which end to aim with. Then there was the hour and a half of dry heaving, until every muscle that could still work felt as if it had been wrung out by the hands of an invisible giant. I knew I had to do something, and like a true addict, the only thing that occurred to me was a falsehood, a mere gesture. I would haul out my briefcase and get the number of my employee assistance plan. I'd go to rehab. That would show my husband and his friends, as well as my employer. I'd show them that *I knew* what they knew, that I knew I had a problem, and that I needed help. And I was going to get it. I'd show them.

Six years later—six years during which I completed one year of twice-weekly outpatient rehab and nightly attendance at twelve-step meetings, and six years during which I remained abstinent—I relapsed. In the meantime, my sons had grown up and all but moved out. We had made a "family geographic," moving from New York to Nevada to be near my sister and to take advantage of the cheaper cost of living in the booming desert. I had made a halfhearted attempt to find a twelve-step meeting near my new home in Las Vegas. After calling the number in the phone book once again, I went to an open meeting in the middle of the day, where I found myself sitting across a table from a man with a disfigured face. When he shared, he talked about losing his nose to his coke addiction. I raced home from the meeting and told my then-still-resident-if-no-longer-quite-faithful husband, "These Las Vegas meetings are too rough and tough for me. I'm doing okay. I haven't had a drink in almost seven years. I'll be all right on my own."

Within a year, my husband had moved in with the woman who would become his second wife, and I was alone in our big, new, empty house. In another couple of months, I was smoking pot. In another month or two, I was drinking harder than I'd ever been. I was a sharply drawn example of the progressive nature of my disease. My alcohol consumption resumed, with greater quantities than ever before, and it just grew and grew, and finally exploded as I married my second husband, a man who was intelligent, handsome, sexy, funny, and completely addicted. That marriage was destined to last only five years.

It was alcohol that had put me on the bathroom floor at the age of seven, and alcohol that found me straddling my second husband's corpse, in a pool of blood, at the age of fifty, slapping his lifeless face as hard as I could, and screaming his name at the top of my lungs. His stomach had virtually exploded from his disease, and for years afterward I lived with the knowledge that for the last four years of his life I had bought, paid for, and brought home every drop of whiskey and beer that he literally lived and died for. As long as he was drinking, I could drink, too. I didn't have to look at myself or my addiction too closely. I didn't have to stop. Until, one day, I did.

One Saturday, just about two years after my second husband died, two long years during which I got a lot of drinking done behind the excuse that I was a desperately unhappy widow, I was shopping in my local market with my two-year-old granddaughter seated in the basket of my shopping cart. As I wheeled her through the liquor aisle, loading my cart with an eighteen-can case of beer and the whiskey that comes in the big brown bottle with the handle, she looked at me with her beautiful, brown, teddy-bear eyes and clearly and distinctly said, "Grannie Hellie, you drink too much whiskey and too much beer."

She was not the first person to make that observation, but she was the one I heard, and maybe the only one I was capable of hearing.

So began my second trip to recovery. I called the number I found in the phone book once again, I got a meeting schedule, and I drove around town looking for the meeting places it listed. Three months after that moment of truth in the supermarket, two and a half years after my second husband died in my arms, eight years after my first marriage was destroyed, I staggered back into the rooms of recovery. Without realizing that's what I was doing, I began to do *The Soul Workout* as if my life depended on it. Because this time, I knew it did.

I've heard it said by many that twelve-step recovery sounds like such a great way of life—what a wonderful world this would be if everyone lived according to these principles. I agree; but I also believe that no one will try to live this way unless the alternative is very clear—"jails, institutions, or death." I've never been in jail (yet), but I've been in institutions, and death will come for me, too, one day, as it will for us all. Death is not what I fear today; a life lived without spiritual values is.

Don't wait until it's too late;
tell those you love that you love them,
every day, while they're here.

Ever notice that if you treat a child badly,
his or her parents don't like you much?
Treat God's other kids nicely—that's the
surest way to a good relationship with God.

**Identify something that you know you
need to change about yourself.**
Are you ready to make that change?
If yes, what do you need to do to start?
If no, what needs to happen
in order for you to be ready?
Remember:
There's no good way to do a bad thing
and no bad way to do a good one.

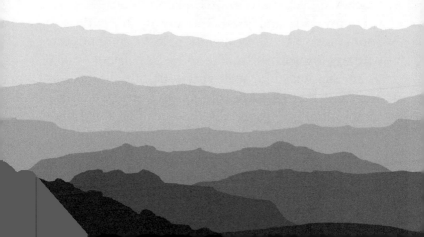

GRATITUDE

Mending My Spirit

One of the spiritual principles my program has instilled in me is gratitude. Every evening, before I go to bed, I try to write a gratitude list of no fewer than five things I've been grateful for that day. On difficult days, the only thing I think I have to be grateful for is the ability to hold a pen. Other times, I have a hard time whittling my list down to just five items. I've come to realize I have much to be grateful for, and cultivating gratitude is a surefire antidote to the impatience and discontent that mark my disease. The two states—gratitude and ingratitude—cannot coexist, and I choose to live in gratitude, with the help of my sponsor, my fellowship, and my Higher Power.

One of the things I'm most grateful for today is the Internet. It was through the Internet that I met Roger, the man I've realized is the love of my life. I keep in touch with my far-flung friends and cousins, learn what my kids and grandkids are up to, and, as a bonus, today I am frequently able to communicate with my former husband, too. The Internet allows me to interact with him with very little of the rancor or bitterness that characterized most of our face-to-face communications, especially the ones that took place toward the end of our marriage.

On a social-networking site we both visit, Sal recently posted that he and his wife were planning to sell their house and leave Las Vegas, where he, she, and I were then living our separate lives. In the subsequent months, I followed with interest his postings as he and Carla endured the challenges of selling a house and buying a new one during a recession. I realized I had sympathy for him and her, which made me feel good about myself. On the other hand, I had to face certain unpleasant truths about myself as well, which surprised me. After all, Sal and I had been divorced for at least ten years by this time. Not only that; he was not the only one to have remarried, and while *his* new wife was alive and well and they were happy together, my second husband had died a horrific death, and I had loved him, grieved him, drunk over his death, and finally entered recovery. As far as my feelings for Sal went, I was so "over him." Wasn't I? Or if I wasn't, shouldn't I have been?

The answer is, as it turns out, yes and no.

The news that Sal and Carla were planning to buy a home in a distant state, in a bucolic, woodsy area, affected me more than I'd thought it would. Memories of the way Sal had always longed to live in the woods flooded back. He had had this dream from the time when we were young together. Well, it seemed that now his wish would be coming true, and it would be coming true with *her*. Not *me*!

Never mind that long ago, during the early years of our difficult marriage, whenever he mentioned this dream of his—to live far away from society, in natural surroundings, far from a city—I would become filled with a sudden and incomprehensible sense of dread. Never mind that he and I could have been the template for "irreconcilable differences" long, long before the state of Nevada dissolved our marriage. Never mind that the thought of living in the woods with him for the rest of my days was and had always been as appealing to me as the idea of being buried alive in a lead-lined coffin. At sea. Never mind any of that. He was doing the thing he'd wanted to do his whole life and he was doing it with *her*! Worse than that, he was doing it without *me*! After divorcing and then living apart from him for ten very eventful years, and after several years in active recovery, I was still capable of dismay that I no longer mattered in his life. Clearly, I had some spiritual housecleaning to do.

First, I had to remember that not only were we divorced, but it was I who had divorced him, that is, once he informed me of his involvement with her. At the time of our breakup I was laid waste, yet I managed to gather myself together sufficiently to enter a second marriage that only ended due to the death of my second husband. It was only after I entered recovery and began working with my sponsor that I began to see my part in these things clearly. Only then could I begin to accept responsibility for my own life and stop blaming others for my suffering.

I remember the beginning of my relationship with my sponsor, Joyce, which started when I was "still bleeding," as they say in my fellowship. She listened patiently as I wailed out my story and heard me out as, whining and moaning, I got to the part about how, six years after I had quit drinking for the first time, my first husband was still evidently unhappy with me and took up with the woman who would become his second wife. My sponsor listened, bemused.

"Wow," she said, dripping irony. "What a creep he was, to try to get a little happiness out of his one and only life."

You have heard the expression "hopping mad"? It almost begins to describe my reaction. I believe I spluttered out the words, "Whose sponsor ARE you?" Joyce knew better than to take offense; after all, she was teaching me. Thus, I began my journey of self-discovery and of learning to look both for and at my part in events and situations that troubled me. I have learned that for many years, during and after my first marriage, it was easier to both rely on and blame Sal for my triumphs and troubles. Now, years after that marriage ended, and having worked a program of recovery for several years, I am just about able to realize that I need to be willing to let go of all my feelings toward him—the good and the bad—if I am ever to be truly free and spiritually fit. I prayed in earnest, "God, remove these feelings from me and direct my attention to what You would have me be." I prayed for patience and for good things for my ex-husband and his wife. I prayed for their happiness and well-being. To stay on my journey of recovery, I worked a Fourth Step on the relationship and moved on to make amends.

One way of making amends to Sal was to try to help him professionally. We had both worked in the publishing field while we were married and both still badly needed freelance gigs, and to this end, I discussed my current job with him. With an eye to offering some work to him, and using the social-networking site we both frequented, I mentioned that I was working on this book.

"YOU are writing a book on spirituality?" he wrote back. I believe he used solid caps.

I understood where he was coming from, and I laughed to myself. Sal and I had both been raised Roman Catholic. While he had completely repudiated that religion by the time we were married in a Gothic Roman Catholic church with bright red doors during a full nuptial Mass in 1972, I had clung, fitfully and fearfully, to vestiges of my childhood faith throughout most of my life. Because of my superstitious fears, we had all of our children baptized in the church.

There came a time, after many years together, when Sal began to explore alternative forms of spirituality, all of which frightened and upset me. I rejected them, and in doing so, made him feel rejected, as I see it now. I remember one particularly vicious exchange regarding his newfound interest in the paranormal:

Sal: "You are SO closed-minded."

Me: "Yeah, and you're so open-minded your brain fell out."

Nice.

Why was I then so surprised when he found a sympathetic and attractive woman who shared his values and beliefs, as I clearly did not?

Sal was within his rights to be skeptical as I sketched out the theme of this book, and told him the title. I touched on some of the exercises to help him understand the sort of book it was.

"*The Soul Workout*?" he teased. "Sounds more like 'The Common Courtesy Workout' to me."

I didn't argue with him. I have learned some things since our divorce, after all. Instead, I thought about what he'd said. I found I agreed with him in large measure. The exercises of *The Soul Workout* amount to thinking of others, sometimes before thinking of one's own wishes, and isn't that the basis of common courtesy?

What is common courtesy, if not, at least in part, taking action against one's own selfish interest? In meetings of my twelve-step fellowship I have heard, over and over again, that the beginning of recovery came when members first began to take actions they didn't think would work, which included, for some, praying to a God they didn't believe in. Often, these actions amount to denying one's own immediate wishes in order to be of service to others, to consider others' feelings above one's own, which is the basis of common courtesy, or what some people call The Golden Rule. Once one takes the right actions, results follow. For me, these have often been quite good results. That is the essence of *The Soul Workout*.

"Good thoughts and good actions cannot have bad results." "I can't think myself into right action, but I can act myself into right thinking." These sentiments infuse the exercises of *The Soul Workout*. Action is the way I express my inward state. Taking actions that cause me a small amount of discomfort, inconvenience, or delay and that take some effort I'd really rather not expend in order to make someone else's life easier—if done with mindfulness, gratitude, and good intent—can help enlarge one's spiritual life. At least it has mine.

Sal would not have used words like "kind," "tolerant," "patient," "loving," or "considerate" to describe the woman he was married to for so many years, so long ago. Yet those are some of the words routinely used to describe me today. Those qualities of kindness, tolerance, patience, love, and consideration all come from within, from my soul. They flow through me, not from me, but they are increasingly powerful the longer I'm in recovery and actively working the principles and steps of the program. My soul has been enlarged. The bigger the soul, the more strength it has and the more of all the positive qualities it can express. How can one gain this strength? Paradoxically, I gained it by practicing those very qualities, even before I fully understood them. It's an endless loop of spirituality and growth.

Do I do this perfectly? No. I don't even manage to practice *The Soul Workout* consistently, much less perfectly. There are days when I am mired in self— self-will, self-centeredness, and selfishness. That's when I need to pause, take a moment, and reach out to others. I need to take a leap beyond the walls of self, take a deep breath, become centered, remember to go to a place of love, and put myself in another's shoes. That's when I need to try to understand, rather than to be understood. I need to remember that place of darkness and despair that I came from and to remember that as dark as it was, there was a dawn. That dawn was of another person holding out her hand to me as she helped me to step into the light. Someone else practicing the principles of *The Soul Workout* showed me that there was indeed light, love, and an awakening to the possibilities within myself. It was then my turn to extend my hand to those around me who also might be having a difficult day, week, or life. By reaching out to others with love and tolerance, and awareness that they, too, might be suffering, I heal and grow my own soul.

I've learned these *Soul Workout* lessons from the members of my fellowship and from people outside my fellowship as well. Everything I've experienced, whether it's been something that's happened to me or something I've accomplished or lost, has served me as a stepping-stone. My experiences allow me to continue the journey I began so very long ago to develop my soul and to continue that journey into the light, more awake and aware that the connection with my Higher Power, which I have always longed for, is within my reach. However, I must reach out. I must take right action. The door to future growth is opening for me, and I joyfully walk through it and into a future filled with more growth, more love, and a more fully developed spirit, able to love and be loved by God's kids and to have a relationship with Him, which, for me, is the ultimate goal of *The Soul Workout*.

My childhood religion taught me that my purpose in this world is to know, love, and serve God. It seems to me today that my program of recovery teaches me the same thing. I grow in knowledge, love, and service to God as I understand Him by means of prayer, meditation, and being of service to Him by serving His other children. Perhaps it's really true that "the more things change, the more they stay the same." The principles I practice today when I do *The Soul Workout* are not new; they are timeless and universal. It's my appreciation of them that is a new thing.

THE SOUL WORKOUT

Put back your shopping cart.
Think about how upset you'd be if you
came out of the supermarket to find your
car dinged by a runaway cart.

Every day identify at least one thing,
however small it may be,
that **you are grateful for.**

If you don't remember someone's name,
rather than pretending that you do, just say,
"Please tell me your name again."
Then repeat it back to them and smile.

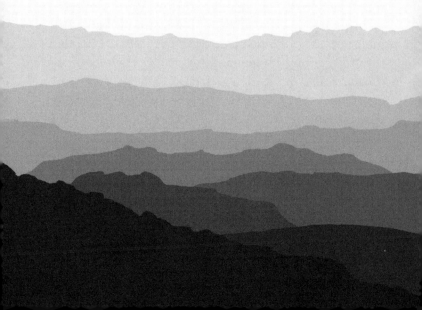

WHAT I "CAME TO BELIEVE"

Opening My Cage

I entered recovery on May 10, and took my first Fifth Step with my sponsor on August 3 of that year. Joyce knew that relief for me would be in the steps, and she didn't let me languish. In fact, as I've learned more about the history of my fellowship during the course of my recovery, I've discovered that in the early days, newcomers were taken through the steps very quickly in order that they might begin their new lives sooner rather than later and begin helping others more quickly.

As part of working Step Two, Joyce asked me about my concept of a Higher Power, and I had to admit, it was a very muddled one. I had discarded or rejected most of my childhood beliefs, which still bedeviled me at times. I had no clear concept of what I wanted the "God of my understanding" to be. Then, one day during this time, as I was trying to write about my beliefs as part of working the Second Step, the image of a golden cage came into my mind. Underneath it, I could see words taking shape: "My God is not a cage." As I meditated on this image, I began to see a little bird inside the cage on a golden perch. Then, as the images became clearer, a golden key appeared and fitted itself into the lock of the cage door, opening it so the bird inside could fly free. The words underneath the image changed: "My God is not a cage; my God is a key," they said. That image helped me greatly in my early recovery.

As time passed, and I practiced *The Soul Workout* without realizing that's what I was doing, I thought about God more and myself less. I began to read recovery literature and talk about God with my sponsor and other fellowship members. Although I've never yet been able to visualize a more "concrete" idea of God, I did begin to formulate some specific ideas about what my God does, even if I don't yet understand quite what my God is.

There's a saying around the meetings of my fellowship: "I am a spiritual being having a human experience." I like that idea and often meditate on it. I now believe that for the past fifty-six years I have been a spiritual being "trapped in the body" of a human. I began to conceive my own "creation myth" about who I am and who my fellow humans are, about why we suffer, and about what the disease of addiction is really all about. I do believe it is a soul sickness that affects my body and mind as well.

My creation myth tells me that when we come into the world, it's God's doing. I imagine that when we are born, He "breaks off" a bit of Himself and puts it into each of us. That's the part we call our souls. Just as when we are born our physical bodies cry the moment we are separated from our mothers, our souls star* crying for reunion with God. The more separate we become from God, the louder the crying gets.

For me, that crying got louder and louder, and I tried to drown it out with alcohol and other drugs. For a while the crying was muffled, but not for long. The crying for God can only be quelled by reunion with God. Many people try stuffing money, sex, food, relationships, or all sorts of things into themselves to quiet that awful crying. The only thing that will work for me, though, is reunion with God. How do I accomplish this? After all, I'm a human being living a human life here on Planet Earth. The way I achieve unity with the God of my understanding is through unity with His other children. How do I accomplish this? By setting aside self and being of service to others; by performing the actions described in this book; by doing *The Soul Workout*.

My God is a key, not a cage. He does not hold me prisoner on an uncomfortable perch.

He opens doors for me and helps me fly.

THE SOUL WORKOUT

As a child, I learned that Christ said, "If anyone desires to come after Me, let him deny himself, and take up his cross daily, and follow me." Maybe we don't have to take up a "cross," but **we can deny ourselves in small ways for others to benefit.** At a birthday party, I can pass the cake instead of taking the biggest piece.

At the market, leave space between yourself and the person on line in front of you (even if they have twelve items in the ten-items-or-fewer aisle). Similarly, let a car trying to enter your lane of traffic pull out in front of you.

Live like a good tenant who is asked to house-sit a mansion. (Because that's actually what you are.) Don't treat your body or your life like a rock star in a hotel room.